The Handbook of Psy[chology for] Forensic Practitioners

The Handbook of Psychology for Forensic Practitioners discusses some of the ways in which psychological research and methods can be applied by a wide variety of professional groups working with offenders. By aiming to give a fuller understanding of how psychology can contribute to our understanding of offending, the book concentrates on the assessment of risk in forensic settings and the interventions designed to reduce risk in violent and sexual offenders.

The book is divided into three parts. The first part includes an overview of major psychological perspectives on offending and this is followed by chapters on the contribution of psychological development and offender profiling. Part II focuses on the assessment of risk with particular emphasis given to two examples: the assessment of risk of suicidal behaviour and violence. Part III looks at the application of psychological assessment and intervention approaches. The focus throughout this section is on the use of systematic approaches to assessment and intervention and the two areas discussed in detail are anger management difficulties and sexual offending.

By illustrating theoretical practice with case examples and also practical guidance *The Handbook of Psychology for Forensic Practitioners* develops a very practical focus throughout the text. It can be used as an aid to day-to-day professional practice for those working in forensic settings including probation officers, social workers, nurses, psychologists and psychiatrists.

Graham J. Towl is Head of Forensic Psychology, East Anglia Area, HM Prison Service and visiting scholar at the University of Cambridge; **David A. Crighton** is a Forensic Psychologist, Yorkshire Centre for Forensic Psychiatry.

The Handbook of Psychology for Forensic Practitioners

Graham J. Towl and
David A. Crighton

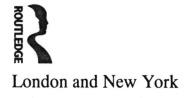

London and New York

Acknowledgements

We would like to thank Jo Bailey for typing a number of the chapters. We would also like to record our appreciation of the sterling work of Adrian Needs in critically commenting on earlier draft chapters of this book. We believe that the quality of the material contained within has improved as a direct result of his comments. Needless to say we take full responsibility for any inaccuracies in the book.

First published 1996
by Routledge
2 Park Square, Milton Park, Abingdon, Oxon, OX14 4RN

Simultaneously published in the USA and Canada
by Routledge
270 Madison Ave, New York NY 10016

Transferred to Digital Printing 2006

© 1996 Graham J. Towl and David A. Crighton

Typeset in Times by
Ponting–Green Publishing Services, Chesham, Bucks

British Library Cataloguing in Publication Data
A catalogue record for this book is available from the
British Library

Library of Congress Cataloguing in Publication Data
A catalogue record for this book has been requested

ISBN 0–415–12887–0 (hbk)
ISBN 0–415–12888–9 (pbk)

Publisher's Note
The publisher has gone to great lengths to ensure the quality of this reprint
but points out that some imperfections in the original may be apparent

Contents

Illustrations

Foreword

Forensic psychology is an expanding field. Every year, more and more psychologists are recruited to work with offenders and other persons showing 'challenging behaviour', to try to help them become more social and better adjusted. Few psychologists believe that 'nothing works', and indeed there is a great deal of recent evidence showing which types of intervention are effective with which types of clients.

The authors of this book have a great deal of experience of working with offenders. Graham Towl is the Head of Psychological Services for HM Prison Service (East Anglia). David Crighton is a forensic psychologist in the National Health Service, working for a regional forensic psychology service. It is remarkable, and a great tribute to their determination, that two busy practitioners have managed to find the time to write a book such as this.

The book is intended as a practical introduction to some aspects of forensic psychology for those who want to find out more about this field. It should be of interest to many, including criminal and civil justice practitioners, probation officers, magistrates, police officers, lawyers, prison staff, forensic psychologists and psychiatrists, social workers, clinical psychologists, criminologists, postgraduate students, policy makers and intelligent lay persons. This book communicates the work of British forensic psychologists to a wide audience.

The first two chapters provide an introductory review of knowledge about offenders gained in psychological research. Chapter 3 reviews the important new field of offender profiling. The authors are perhaps a little more critical than I would be, but it is essential to draw attention to the problems of any new technique that need to be overcome in the future. Chapters 4 to 6 provide extremely valuable practical information on risk assessment, focusing on the areas of suicide and violence. Chapters 7 to 9 focus on cognitive–behavioural approaches to anger management techniques using group work. Chapters 10 to 12 provide insightful reviews of knowledge about sex offenders and techniques for assessment and treatment.

The authors succeed in distilling practical skills and experience for the benefit of a wide audience. The book constitutes an important 'how to do it' manual of techniques for risk assessment, anger management and sex offender treatment. In the light of the current significance of all three topics, and the importance of future workers building on the experience and knowledge of past workers, I am very happy to welcome this book and recommend it as a scholarly and highly readable introduction to some key areas of work undertaken by forensic psychologists.

David P. Farrington
Professor of Psychological Criminology
Cambridge University

Introduction

For expository purposes this handbook is divided into three parts: (1) offenders; (2) risk assessment; (3) interventions. Our aims in writing this book are to provide forensic practitioners from a range of disciplines with:

1 A fuller understanding of psychological contributions to what we know about offenders.
2 A framework for undertaking risk assessment work.
3 Intervention strategies for working with offenders with anger management difficulties.
4 Intervention strategies for working with sex offenders.

These aims reflect a necessarily selective set of areas relevant to forensic practitioners. However, from our examination of the literature in the field and discussions with a broad range of colleagues in the forensic field it is evident to us that the areas covered will be of interest and relevance to practitioners from a range of professional backgrounds.

The first part of the book, on offenders, is intended to provide information on psychological contributions to our general understanding of offenders. The next part of the book, on risk assessment, begins with an outline of a generic framework for structuring risk assessments in forensic practice. The framework is applied in two subsequent chapters on suicide and violence. Our third and final part covers two areas – anger management and sex offender interventions. We could have chosen a number of other areas to illustrate psychological contributions to forensic practice; these two were chosen because of the widespread growth and relevance of such work in a range of forensic settings (e.g. in prisons, special hospitals, regional secure units and with offenders on probation orders). Inevitably the inclusion of some areas will result in the exclusion of others. We make no claims of comprehensive coverage of the forensic field, this would be a mammoth task well beyond the aims of this book.

We begin with a general overview of major psychological perspectives. The contributions of some key studies in developmental and social psychology in particular are outlined in terms of their potential relevance for forensic practitioners. Theories of both intellectual and moral development are critically examined in relation to their implications for our understanding of offenders. Areas of social psychology addressed include: attitudes, attribution theory, cognitive dissonance and group processes. We contend that an understanding of such core social psychological processes is helpful in understanding the behaviour of offenders. The second chapter further develops some of the developmental themes from the first, drawing heavily upon what has become known as 'criminal career' research studies. Such studies have produced much information about offenders which has, particularly in recent years, represented one of the major contributions to criminological psychology.

The third chapter in this section covers offender profiling. We argue that despite the media attention and research efforts in this area the results of such work have been overwhelmingly disappointing to date. However, it is an important area to consider as a recent development in forensic psychology. The area does hold the potential to help further develop our understanding of offenders and crime. We would argue that the research in this area could perhaps most usefully be taken forward by a further integration of ideas across other rich sources of our knowledge base about offenders (e.g. insights derived from developmental and social psychology).

Part II, on risk assessment, includes consideration of conceptual and practice difficulties associated with undertaking such work. We outline and propose a generic framework for forensic practitioners to help inform effective practice. We maintain that the term 'risk' is best used as a statement of probability followed by a clear specification of target behaviours that we are trying to estimate the risk of occurring. We highlight the importance of identifying not only factors which would increase the risk of, say, reoffending but also factors which would decrease the level of risk.

In Chapter 6, we acknowledge that much violence, for example, corporate violence, may be very harmful indeed. However, it is comparatively rare for perpetrators of such violence to have any involvement with the criminal or civil justice system. For this reason we focus our discussion on violence chiefly in three areas: murder, assaults and robbery. Practitioners in the criminal justice system will undoubtedly encounter clients who have offended in at least one of these categories. We examine the psychological and social context of such crimes. Also, we attempt to illustrate how our framework for risk assessment may be applied in the prediction of violent offending.

In the third part of this book we focus on intervention work. We begin the section with a chapter on cognitive–behavioural approaches to intervention. We include a brief history of the background to such approaches. The techniques covered may be applied to a range of difficulties experienced by offenders. However, there remains much work to be done in further developing such interventions. We believe that cognitive–behavioural approaches to interventions with offenders will remain at the forefront of effective work with offenders for some years to come.

In Chapter 8 we give some guidelines on how the practitioner may make an assessment of the anger management difficulties of offenders. In recent years interest in anger management interventions, largely based upon the influential work of Raymond Novaco, appears to have increased considerably. Despite such interest, there remains some confusion about differences and links between anger and aggression. Indeed, we believe that one of the main reasons for the expansion of such work has been based on the belief that there is a direct link between anger and aggression. We address these issues more fully in the assessment chapter. In Chapter 9, the treatment of anger management difficulties, we outline an example of a programme of groupwork to address anger management difficulties. The treatment programme is structured to cover an example of possible content materials but also, and most importantly, we address process issues. Content and process issues are covered in terms of aims and objectives for each session. In considering this area we prefer the use of the term anger management rather than anger control. This is because the term 'anger control' often may give offenders the impression that they simply have to 'overcontrol' their anger and indeed be passive in their behaviour when angry. The term 'management' seems to us to lend itself more readily to a broader consideration of methods of channelling and expressing anger. Indeed, one of the key themes in such work involves the distinction between the experience and expression of anger.

Chapter 10 provides a summary of what we know about sex offenders. We outline some approaches to categorising such offences. We then go on to consider rape and child molesting, both within and outwith the family, in greater detail. We advocate the use of the term 'child molesting' in preference to the term 'paedophile', since the latter means 'lover of children'. This seems to us a very misleading term for offenders who sexually assault children.

Chapter 11 provides an illustration of the cognitive–behavioural approach to assessing sex offenders. We include practical advice on how to conduct assessment interviews and what further information practitioners need to glean from other sources. Assessments based on the methods we outline will, we believe, be helpful to practitioners faced with addressing appropriate treatment interventions. We emphasise the importance of accurate assessment and its link to appropriate treatment.

Chapter 12 is on the treatment of sex offenders. We adopt precisely the same approach to structuring this work as for the treatment of anger management in Chapter 9. This is because we feel that the same general cognitive–behavioural principles apply across a range of intervention areas. Also, we believe that consistency of approach is helpful to good practice. In undertaking treatment work we advocate wherever possible the use of group-based approaches with sex offenders as a more effective intervention strategy. We also consistently try to emphasise the importance of treatment as a way to reduce the risk of further offending. In common with our views on other areas of treatment and risk assessment we see the use of effective monitoring and support as an essential and ongoing part of an effective approach.

We have written this handbook for practitioners to draw from in their day-to-day work. As such, some chapters are likely to be of greater interest to some practitoners. Each chapter though can be read as a guide to practice in its own right. This inevitably means that we have at times reiterated information.

We hope that this book will serve as a useful tool for forensic practitioners and hope that most readers will find something useful for their practice in these pages.

Graham Towl and David Crighton
December 1995

Part I

What we know about offenders

Chapter 1

What we know about offenders

An overview of major psychological perspectives

INTRODUCTION

Psychology is not the only discipline to be concerned with understanding criminal and delinquent behaviour. Indeed, disciplines such as social policy, sociology and criminology have traditionally been far more central to the study of this area than psychology. Historically there have sometimes been inherent tensions between these disciplines and psychological approaches. This seems to have been largely because the approaches of psychologists were seen as locating the causes of criminality within the individual, at the expense of attending to the effects of social inequalities. This is seen in much psychological research. Other disciplines, for example, sociology, have perhaps been slow to accept and address the effects of individual differences in the face of similar social conditions.

However, it seems that in recent years there has been a greater degree of overlap between psychological approaches and other social science disciplines than ever before. This is, we would argue, due to an opening up of psychological approaches to encompass real-world rather than laboratory-based problems. This has, it seems, brought psychologists much closer in some areas to the views of other social scientists. Much of the recent work in developmental and social psychology has demonstrated the very powerful influences that both social inequalities and social environments can have on people's behaviour.

Equally some areas of study in psychology have overlapped with the biological sciences. This has led to an interest in biological differences between people and the effects of these on behaviour. A great deal of research has been undertaken into the biological correlates of offending and delinquency. We discuss these in greater detail below. It is probably fair to say that this aspect of psychological research has been extremely controversial. It is also an approach which has often antagonised other social scientists. Many have seen such approaches as being politically dangerous. Genetics-based research has often been associated with extreme right-wing political views. Concerns have been expressed about the potential dangers in such research, for example, the development of policies based on naive and simplistic ideas about biological differences (see Rose *et al.*, 1984). Research concerned with environmental influences in contrast has often been associated with left-wing politics.

We would acknowledge these concerns fully. We review this area of research below. What seems clear from this research is that there is a very great deal of variation between people in terms of biological factors; everything from height to patterns of brain activity in fact. However, the implications of this variation are by no means fully understood. Whilst small sub-groups of offenders do appear to suffer from neurological abnormalities the vast majority do not. Even here it is not clear whether these biological differences are a cause or a consequence of their behaviour. The idea that there is any single explanation of complex behaviours is logically untenable. Crime covers a huge range of possible behaviours. Crime is also a social construct which changes over time and across cultures, in that each society will decide what behaviours should and should not be proscribed. It also seems clear that criminal justice systems appear to often work inequitably across social and economic groups.

It would be naive to assume that 'scientific' research in the behavioural sciences can be objective in the sense of being removed from the social and political context; sadly this is a view propounded (often implicitly) by some researchers. Below we outline a number of psychological perspectives on offending based on empirical research.

THE CONTRIBUTION OF DEVELOPMENTAL PSYCHOLOGY

Developmental psychology has traditionally been concerned with the development of an individual from conception to adulthood and how this relates to their psychological functioning. More recently, developmental psychology has expanded to include the notion of lifespan development. As such, developmental psychology is fundamental to an adequate understanding of criminal and delinquent behaviour. In particular we would suggest that an understanding of social, personality and intellectual development is crucial.

It seems clear from the existing research that intellectual development is greatly influenced by a child's environment. These influences can begin well before birth in terms of effects on later intellectual functioning. In this respect, those from more economically deprived backgrounds tend to fare worse. A clear example of this is the fact that those living in economically deprived inner city areas in industrialised societies tend to be exposed to higher levels of lead pollution (mainly from petrol fumes and lead water pipes). Lead has been shown to cause neurological damage which in turn is associated with lower IQ scores (Bellinger *et al.*, 1991). This is just one example of the damaging effects of a poor environment.

Parenting styles have also been shown to have a major impact on later behaviour. Whilst there is some evidence that children differ markedly in their behaviour at birth (Chess and Thomas, 1984) this is strongly shaped by parental behaviours. Some styles of parenting appear to be much more successful in developing good levels of self-esteem in a child, as well as characteristics such as empathy for and altruism towards others. Children who show later problem behaviours such as aggression towards others tend to come, disproportionately, from families which show inconsistent discipline, rejection and the use of harsh punishments (Eron *et al.*, 1991).

Another area of developmental psychology which we would suggest is particularly important in understanding criminal and delinquent behaviour is the study of development during adolescence. This is an age where the frequency and severity of delinquent behaviours increases markedly. It is also when the majority of offenders will have their first contacts with the police. There is good evidence that there are consistent aspects of a person's background which will largely predict who will get into such trouble (see Farrington, 1991). There would appear to be a variety of factors involved in why adolescence is linked to a peak in such behaviours. It is the time when children begin to mature into adults and go through the changes of puberty. Adolescents also spend more time away from their homes and families and with peer groups. A large amount of offending seen at this age appears to involve groups rather than individuals. In the United States the arrest rate for those aged between 15 and 17 years is about 11 per cent of the age group. The proportion is much higher for those living in economically deprived areas. The majority of these arrests tend to be for acts such as shoplifting, vandalism and illegal use of alcohol, although about a third related to felonies (i.e. crimes such as burglary, rape, arson and murder) (Dryfoos, 1990). The Cambridge study found similarly high rates of offending and even higher rates of self-reported delinquent behaviours (Farrington, 1991).

Another very significant aspect of developmental psychology thought to be particularly relevant to offending and delinquency has been the study of moral reasoning. This derives largely from the work of psychologists who initially began studying intellectual development in young children. The most influential work in this respect has perhaps been that of Kohlberg (1964). Kohlberg suggested that an individual's ability to reason about moral matters develops in stages, analogous to stage theories of general intellectual development. This is an area which we develop further in Chapter 2.

THE CONTRIBUTION OF SOCIAL PSYCHOLOGY

Social psychology can be defined as the scientific study of social behaviour (Aronson, 1972). Social behaviour includes everything from brief interactions between two people through to complex interaction between groups of people. Since people are very much social beings, this means that social psychology covers a huge range of behaviours. Everything from interpersonal attraction and romantic love to racial hatred and violence. Clearly this means that in discussing the impact of this area of psychology to our understanding of crime and crime-related behaviours we can only summarise a few key areas of research in social psychology. There are some areas of social psychology which we would suggest have been particularly relevant and valuable in furnishing us with insights into offending and delinquent behaviour. Below we outline some of these areas.

ATTITUDES AND BEHAVIOUR

The study of attitudes in social psychology has largely focused on what people say when asked about particular subjects, and how these expressed attitudes influence their actual behaviour. Interestingly, the early research into attitudes suggested that there was a poor relationship between attitudes and behaviours. Wicker (1969) concluded that only in a minority of cases was a close relationship found between expressed attitudes and behaviour. Indeed there have been several studies which clearly showed people acting in contradiction of their expressed attitudes. An example of this was a study conducted by LaPierre in 1934 in the United States. Following a questionnaire to restaurant owners concerning their attitudes about 'the Chinese race', LaPierre visited these establishments. Despite the fact that nearly all those questioned had expressed anti-Chinese attitudes, none of the restaurants in fact failed to serve LaPierre and his two Chinese confederates.

The reasons for this apparent paradox between what people say and what they do seems to be due, in large part to the way these studies were conducted. In most early studies very general measures of attitudes were taken and compared with very specific measures of behaviour (Ajzen and Fishbein, 1977). In this early study the researchers failed to ask restaurant owners about their likely behaviours, as well as their attitudes. More recent research suggests that the decision by an individual about whether to act on the basis of an attitude will depend on a complex decision-making process. This will include both an evaluation of their own behaviour and consideration of the likely evaluations of others (Fishbein, 1967). In the example of the restaurateurs given above the views of other customers would be relevant. This complex link between attitudes and behaviours is of clear relevance to many offenders. As we will discuss in greater detail a proportion of violent offenders may evaluate their own worth in terms of their ability and willingness to be violent towards others, and similarly may value the views of their peer group who they believe (often correctly) will similarly value such behaviour. Other offenders may find ways of avoiding the likely negative evaluations of others. So, for example, child molesters often go to great lengths to keep their behaviour secret, or to associate with others who will support their attitudes.

In terms of working with offenders the research into attitudes and behaviour is important. This is not least because it draws into question the value of general measures of attitudes among offenders as predictors of behaviour. This area of research also highlights the importance of situational constraints in shaping how an individual will react.

ATTRIBUTION THEORIES

This area of research derives mainly from the work of Heider (1944; 1958). Attribution theories are concerned with how people ascribe causes to particular behaviours. Examples of this would include a wide variety of 'personality attributions'. For example, someone might be described as being extrovert (meaning that they are confident, outgoing and sociable). Similar personality attributions are also often made in forensic settings, and terms such as 'manipulative' are examples of such character attributions about behaviour. The assumptions behind such an attribution are that the person is choosing to behave in this way and has the option to behave in other ways. We cover this area in greater detail when we discuss the risk of suicidal behaviour in Chapter 5.

However, there appears to be a fundamental tendency among people to consistently underestimate the impact of situational conditions; and also to overestimate the impact of dispositional factors. Heider suggested that this was because of a fundamental human tendency to focus on the behaviour observed and fail to pay enough attention to the context in which the behaviour takes place (Heider, 1958).

Kelley (1967; 1971) looked at such attributions and produced an explanatory model for how we go about making attributions about the causes of other people's behaviour. In this model he suggested that the attributions we make depend on three main factors: firstly, how distinctive a particular behaviour is; secondly, how consistent it is over time; thirdly, the degree of consensus about how appropriate the behaviour is. So, for example, where an individual showed a very distinctive behaviour consistently over time, and there was low consensus about this behaviour, we would tend to make dispositional attributions. An example of this might be an individual who severely assaulted people whom he thought were laughing at him in the pub. Here, this is generally a distinctive behaviour in most public houses. It is being consistently shown by this person, and in this example most people would not accept the motivation as reasonable. Thus, the consensus for the behaviour is low. In this case most people would make a dispositional attribution.

One problem with this model is that it is rarely that we can make decisions on the basis of having all this information available. It also seems to be the case that people do not make the best logical use of the information available in the way suggested by the model. Certain systematic biases appear to occur in making attributions about the behaviour of others. One of the most significant systematic biases is the failure to take into account base-rate information, i.e. how often a behaviour occurs in the population. Experimental studies suggest that people will generally ignore this information in favour of systematic biases. Indeed, people are very resistant to using base-rate information under any circumstances when making judgements about others (see Kahneman and Tversky, 1973).

A second tendency is that people show a marked preference for making internal or character attributions, even when there is strong evidence to contradict such interpretations. An experimental illustration of the strength of this tendency was given by Jones and Harris (1967). In this study they gave students two essays to read, one favouring the communist revolution in Cuba, one against. Students were asked to listen to these speeches and to rate the presenters in terms of their political views.

Despite the fact that those doing the ratings knew the selection of the essay readers was random, they still rated those who presented the pro-revolution essays as being more left wing in their political views. A more practical example are some cases of suicide in custody where those assessing the person have shown clear evidence of making strong dispositional attributions about the person who committed suicide (i.e. manipulative, attention seeking). This is often done at the expense of situational factors, for example, in the case of teenage boys remanded to large local prisons and lacking any family or social support. Here, there are often clear and strong situational factors which are likely to increase the risk of suicidal and self-harming behaviours. In many cases these seem to be minimised by observing staff in favour of character-based explanations of behaviour (see Chapter 5).

Two other biases in our interpretation of other people's behaviour are of interest. One has been called the actor–observer difference. In brief, those involved in a particular behaviour will rate much more highly the situational factors leading them to behave in particular ways, whilst outside observers will rate dispositional factors much more highly. Another is that there is a greater tendency to make dispositional attributions where the consequences of a behaviour have been more serious (see Jones and Nisbett, 1971).

This would seem to have clear implications for the assessment of risk of reoffending with offenders, especially where the consequences of their behaviour are considered to have been 'serious'. The relevance of such findings to forensic practice is, we would argue, that there is a strong tendency to overvalue dispositional ideas such as a particular client being aggressive, at the expense of situational factors which may, for example, be sustaining the behaviour.

COGNITIVE DISSONANCE

Cognitive dissonance is a theory developed by Festinger (1957). According to this theory any decision between alternative courses of action which are both valued to some degree by the person will lead to a state of psychological tension or 'dissonance'. The level of this dissonance will depend on the degree to which the two choices are similarly attractive to the individual. This state of discomfort does not appear to dissipate immediately a choice is made but will persist whilst the chosen behaviour is taking place. To reduce this state of psychological discomfort the person needs to engage in thinking which increases the attractiveness of the chosen behaviour and decreases the attractiveness of the behaviour not chosen. This process of re-evaluation and selective recall reduces an individual's feelings of psychological discomfort. This is a process which may be seen in offenders.

Bem (1967) developed this idea into what he termed self-perception theory. Attitudinal responses were, he suggested, influenced by processes of self-observation. In this theory he suggests that if we behave in particular ways, we are likely to restructure some of our expressed attitudes to fit with the behaviour (Kiesler *et al.*, 1969). This, however, does not appear to be true of instances where people are forced to behave in particular ways. Here it appears that people simply make situational attributions about their behaviour (e.g. 'I was forced to do it.'). Where these situational factors are absent then we appear to make more dispositional attributions about our own behaviour.

The work on cognitive dissonance perhaps suggests reasons why some offenders invest so much in developing reasons, justifications and explanations for their behaviour. It also suggests ways that these processes could be changed.

GROUP PROCESSES

The study of groups in social psychology is concerned with similar processes but where groups of three or more people are involved. There is a long history in social psychology of studying such behaviour both in terms of within and between group processes.

The power of group processes to influence the behaviour of individuals has been repeatedly demonstrated. For example, Sherif in 1935 showed that group members could be influenced to change their judgements about a visual illusion in the direction of the group consensus. This occurred even where this consensus was extremely inaccurate. Convergence seemed to be greater where the interpersonal relationships among the group were positive (Sampson and Insko, 1964). The adoption of such group norms does not though appear to be as ubiquitous as once thought, and appears to be influenced by factors such as the degree of liking between group members, and the level of perceived uncertainty in the judgements being undertaken.

There may be a high level of group conformity where there is no uncertainty about the judgements being made. Asch (1951; 1956) looked at the degree of group conformity on a simple objective task (i.e. judging which of two lines was longer). Asch found that about one in three people would conform to an incorrect response. This level of conformity though was greatly reduced where there was another group member who gave the correct and non-conforming response. What appears to be important here is that where a group appears to be unanimously opposed to an individual's viewpoint, then the vast majority of individuals will become more uncertain about their own judgements. If an individual's confidence in his or her own judgement is undermined, then many such individuals will respond in accordance with what they think they ought to see. Other studies have suggested that 'deviant' individuals (i.e. those who disagree with the group consensus) will tend to be rejected by the group (Schacter, 1951). Similarly non-conformist group members will tend to hold negative views on those group members who conformed to a false consensus (Gerard and Greenbaum, 1962). Where there is a consistent and non-conformist minority this is not so easy for group members to ignore, and this appears to be more crucial in changing group beliefs than simple numerical superiority.

Whilst these may appear to be, and indeed are, somewhat artificial experimental procedures they do seem to have clear parallels with the effects of groups in more naturalistic settings. Group effects also seem to be important for much offending and delinquent behaviour, particularly in the case of younger offenders. Such research also gives some insight into the group processes which may be helpful in facilitating attitude change.

DEINDIVIDUATION

This is a concept developed by Philip Zimbardo. Zimbardo (1969) based this concept on the assumption that group behaviour can be qualitatively different from individual behaviour. The idea here is that when in a group an individual can operate in a 'deindividuated' manner, showing forms of behaviour that would not otherwise be seen. Although Zimbardo did not suggest that deindividuation was a necessary, or even a sufficient condition, for delinquent behaviours, it does seem to have clear value in contributing to explanations of some types of criminal and violent behaviours.

The processes involved appear to be a minimising of 'self-observation' and concern about social evaluation. This is followed by a weakening of the controls over behaviour such as fear or guilt. In turn this seems to be followed by a lowering of the threshold for displaying otherwise inhibited behaviours. Examples of such deindividuated behaviour might include offences such as gang rapes and gang violence. Other frequently cited and controversial examples include the occurrence of wartime atrocities and the unprofessional behaviour of the police and armed forces during riots or civil disturbances.

The concept is supported by experimental studies in social psychology which have shown that people can behave in uncharacteristically aggressive ways when given conditions which 'deindividuate' them. For example, in a study by Zimbardo (1969) he found that women college students were prepared to administer simulated electric shocks to others at higher intensity when part of a group.

A particularly dramatic study was undertaken by Zimbardo and colleagues in the form of an observational study into prison behaviour (Zimbardo, 1975). In fact the study was funded by the US Navy and the scenario used was more analogous to a prisoner of war camp than to a civilian prison or secure hospital. The study used male students from Stanford University and randomly allocated volunteers to be 'guards' or 'prisoners'. Both groups were given uniforms which were likely to increase the level of deindividuation. This included dark glasses and uniforms for the 'guards' and standard clothing for the 'prisoners'. The results of this study surprised even the researchers. There was a very rapid escalation in the use of arbitrary power and punishments by the 'guards'. Responses from the 'prisoners' ranged from aggression and violence to marked distress. Emotional reactions included depression, crying, rage and acute anxiety.

This was in many respects a flawed study. It is open to question how ethical the behaviour of the researchers was. Others have questioned why the study deviated so far from the regimes of normal civilian prisons, where in most countries prisoners are more clear about the legal processes which govern their custody. This is perhaps because the study more closely paralleled the experience of prisoner of war camps. The escalation of brutality seen here has numerous historical parallels in such camps. However, the results were so dramatic that they cannot be dismissed. The study provides a clear and dramatic illustration of the powerful effects of 'deindividuating' conditions on behaviour.

The study also tells us something about the dangers inherent in custodial institutions. When conducted, the study served a valuable function in the USA by countering the then prevalent dispositional view about prisoners, namely that prisons were violent and brutal places exclusively because that was the nature of the prisoners. Clearly in this case it had been demonstrated that situational conditions could powerfully influence behaviour. The findings of this study are also important in contributing to our understanding of some of the unprofessional behaviour of staff in secure hospitals and prisons.

THE CONTRIBUTION OF BIOLOGICAL PSYCHOLOGY

A number of the research approaches used today in psychology are derived from the biological sciences, and there remain significant areas of overlap between psychology and sciences, such as physiology. Here we look at research which is concerned with the link between biological changes and behaviour.

The idea of any biological links to offending is strongly resisted by many social scientists and also psychologists. It is probably true to state that much of the biological research has become politically tainted. Simple notions about criminal behaviour being inherited, or amenable to physical interventions such as brain surgery are clearly very dangerous and have been associated with extreme right-wing political ideologies (see Rose *et al.*, 1984).

Some early biological approaches (e.g. Lange, 1931) took a very clearly determinist approach, namely that biological defects or deficits led to criminal behaviour. The appalling conclusion of this perverse logic was perhaps best illustrated in the activities of the Nazi regime in 1930s Germany.

Few today would argue in favour of such biological determinism and the currently favoured view in physiological psychology is one of 'biological interactionism'. This is simply the idea that biological processes are shaped by, and interact with, the environment that an individual experiences (Rowe and Osgood, 1984). This would include 'biological environments' such as that experienced by an individual during foetal development. This challenges the notion sometimes portrayed that the environment is exclusively an individual's 'social world'.

What does seem clear from the research is that individuals are not born with equal biological potential and that differences between people are present soon after birth. In a study of newborn infants, Chess and Thomas (1984) found marked differences between the behaviours seen, which in turn went on to predict some later behaviours. Thus, for example, children who were easily upset as newborns tended to continue this pattern into childhood. They argued from their research that parenting was far from being unidirectional, but that the child can greatly influence the behaviour of the parents.

GENETIC RESEARCH

There is an ongoing debate within psychology about the relative impact of heredity and environment on behaviour. What does seem to be agreed though is that both will have some influence. Thus it has been argued that genetic inheritance sets the limits on an individual, whilst it is the environment which influences the expression of those limits. So, for example, individuals may inherit genes to become very tall. However, if they grow up in an environment where they are constantly malnourished, it is unlikely they will attain their full (potential) height. In this example it is clear that the environment has restricted the expression of the individual's genetic potential. Similarly in reverse, someone inheriting genes to be of average height is unlikely to reach a height of, say, 6 feet 5 inches however well fed they are. The analogy between physical and psychological differences is not clear cut though. Physical characteristics such as height or eye colour can be measured with a high degree of accuracy. Measurements of psychological differences are much less precise. These measurements are often assumed to reflect underlying physical differences. It is, though, probably reasonable to state that our understanding of such differences is not adequate to make such a direct link.

Studies of criminal or delinquent behaviour are far from being as clear cut as this simple example. Early studies focused on the fact that criminal behaviour tended to run in families. However, where this is true we would argue that environmental explanations are far more credible and of greater use to forensic practitioners than genetic ones.

More sophisticated studies have looked at identical and non-identical twins who have been separated. One of the earliest such studies was that of Lange (1931) who looked at male twins, claiming that 77 per cent of identical and 12 per cent of non-identical twins had similar criminal histories (called concordance rates). Later studies have agreed with the direction of this finding, but not to the levels reported by Lange. Indeed as studies have become better designed and run, the difference between identical and non-identical twins in terms of offending has reduced (Christiansen, 1977). Another problem with this type of research has been the extent to which pairs of twins were truly brought up separately and so experienced differing environments. So in early studies, for example, there were cases where twins had been raised by mother and grandmother in adjacent houses, but had been classified as separated. Here it seems clear that these twins would experience a very similar environment when growing up (Rose *et al.*, 1984).

In another study Rowe (1983) looked at self-reported delinquent behaviour in twins. In this study high levels of similarity were found for the identical twins. However, the levels for non-identical twins were lower but still high. Whilst this suggests that genetic inheritance may

Table 1.1 Genetic influences on criminal behaviour in twins

	Male (%)	Female (%)
Identical	35	21
Non-identical	13	8

Source: Christiansen 1977
Note: Percentage where both twins had criminal histories

have some influence on later delinquency it is far from being as compelling as early claims about biological influences. Similarly, one of the most recent and authoritative studies of genetic influences on criminal behaviour was conducted by Christiansen (1977) who looked at all the twins in an area of Denmark (3,586 pairs in all). The results of this study are summarised in Table 1.1.

Whilst these results may provide some support for a genetic predisposition, it is much less than has been claimed by some in the past. The results also suggest that more twins behave differently than behave similarly in terms of criminal behaviour, a finding which may in fact provide good evidence for the power of environmental effects.

ADOPTION STUDIES

This type of study has looked at the outcomes of adopted children in comparison to their adoptive and biological parents. The assumption here has been that any observed similarity to biological parents will be inherited. An example of such research is a study by Hutchings and Mednick (1975) again in Denmark. This study looked at 143 adopted children with biological fathers who had criminal records and compared these to 143 adopted children where the biological father had no criminal record. They found that 36 per cent of these boys offended themselves where both biological and adoptive fathers had criminal records; 21 per cent offended where the biological father only had a criminal record; and 10 per cent offended where neither father had a criminal record. The researchers argued that this result was consistent with a genetic effect. However, we would suggest that these results are far from convincing in this respect, and that many of the initial assumptions about the adoptees were potentially misleading. For example, it is unclear to what extent these boys were exposed to criminal fathers as potential role models.

STUDIES OF CHROMOSOMAL ABNORMALITIES

Chromosomal abnormalities are where there are variations from the normal genetic structure of the cells. Perhaps the best-known example of this is Down's syndrome, although there are many more. Interest in a possible link between the occurrence of certain chromosomal abnormalities and offending dates back to the 1960s and focused almost exclusively on abnormalities in the sex chromosome. Several studies have shown an increased incidence of abnormal sex chromosomes in institutionalised patients, although similar abnormalities are found in 0.1 per cent of the general population (Jarvick *et al.*, 1973).

It now seems clear that a wide variety of chromosomal abnormalities are more common in institutions such as secure hospitals and this seems to be strongly linked to lower levels of intellectual functioning. In addition, the occurrence of such disorders is very rare and accounts for only a tiny fraction of criminal behaviour.

PSYCHOPHYSIOLOGICAL RESEARCH

The term psychophysiological is generally used to refer to attempts to measure physical changes in the body in response to psychological events (see Price *et al.*, 1982). A wide range of such measures have been used with forensic populations. Perhaps the best known of these is the electroencephalograph (EEG), which measures electrical activity in the brain. The results of such research have been disappointing in that the reported results have been inconsistent. Some researchers have claimed high levels of abnormal EEGs in aggressive offenders, others have found no difference (Syndulko *et al.*, 1975).

This is perhaps partially explained by the variety of methods used to measure EEGs. In addition, EEG recordings have been demonstrated to be influenced by short-term events in a person's environment, such as boredom. Gendreau *et al.* (1972) found that solitary confinement of prisoners resulted in a slowing of their EEGs. We would argue that it is not hard to see how institutionalised groups of offenders could come to give peculiar EEG readings simply as an effect of the environment they live in and the influence of this on their behaviour.

Mednick *et al.* (1981) conducted one of the few prospective studies into EEG abnormalities and found that boys arrested on two or more occasions did tend to show consistent differences on their EEGs, compared to non-offending boys. Subsequent studies have shown that these patterns are seen in both property and violent offenders and also in a proportion of non-delinquents (Hsu *et al.*, 1985).

Much of this inconsistency may be due to the fact that EEG measures are very global and non-specific measures of brain functioning. This idea led some researchers (e.g. Raine, 1989) to take more specific measures of brain functioning. Here again, whilst some researchers claim to have found identifiable differences in the brain activity of offenders, others have found no clear differences (e.g. Fenton *et al.*, 1978; Hare, 1985; 1986). The issue is also clouded further by the fact that many such studies have looked at 'psychopathic' offenders as a diagnostic category, rather than looking at groups of offenders on the basis of actual offending. Finally, some would question the meaning of any such findings. Whilst most researchers in this area appear to assume that abnormal patterns of brain activity precede, for example, violent offending, it is also plausible that they are after-effects of engaging in such behaviours.

BRAIN DYSFUNCTION AND DELINQUENCY

Rutter (1982) points out that there is no simple relationship between neurological damage and behaviour. It seems clear that severe damage does have a major impact on behaviour. However, children in particular seem in many cases to be able to recover from brain injury. Others will show delinquent behaviour with no evidence of physical pathology. Therefore most studies of delinquency and brain dysfunction have relied on indirect measures such as psychological tests or EEGs, rather than looking at physical measures of brain damage.

An exception to this is epilepsy. It has been estimated that 0.5 per cent of the population suffer from some form of epilepsy. Similar rates have been found in the prison population (Gunn *et al.*, 1991), although the researchers felt this was an underestimate due to methodological limitations in their study.

It has been suggested that temporal lobe epilepsy is associated with abnormally high levels of aggression. The role of parts of the brain close to the temporal lobes in producing 'rage' reactions in both animals and man is well documented (Ganong, 1991). This has led to the suggestion that in some cases non-specific temporal lobe dysfunction may be involved in violence (Monroe, 1978).

Whilst this may be a factor in a comparatively small number of cases it is not the case for the vast majority of aggressive offenders. It is even more problematic where behaviours such as aggression are attributed to a hypothesised neurological disorder which is not directly observable.

The 'explanation' in this instance becomes entirely circular and as such quite unhelpful.

THE CONTRIBUTION OF BEHAVIOURAL PSYCHOLOGY

The behavioural approach to psychology has been the dominant approach for much of the history of modern psychology. Indeed, it is only in recent years that the influence of cognitive approaches has dramatically changed psychology as a research and an applied discipline. Behavioural psychology has had at least two key effects. Firstly, by emphasising the importance of what is observable (i.e. behaviour), it placed a great emphasis on careful analysis, observation and measurement which was largely absent prior to the development of behavioural approaches. This emphasis is generally reflected throughout psychology and also in the applications of psychology to applied problems (see Goldstein and Foa, 1980). Secondly, behavioural approaches emphasised the importance of the testability of any ideas or hypotheses about behaviour against clear behavioural criteria.

One of the legacies of the behavioural approach has been the development of a range of intervention techniques to address particular problem behaviours, these techniques having proven efficacy in modifying particular behaviours. The clearest examples of this would be in the reduction of anxiety or obsessional behaviours (see Hawton *et al.*, 1989).

Despite this, the contributions of behavioural psychology to the understanding of complex behaviours such as delinquency and crime have been rather limited. This has only really changed in recent years with the integration of cognitive and behavioural approaches into a cognitive–behavioural framework. Prior to this attempts were made to explain delinquent behaviours in purely behavioural terms (e.g. Skinner, 1971). However, these were seen by many as fundamentally flawed and unconvincing accounts, not least because they were entirely deterministic. Thus, they accounted for all behaviour entirely in terms of environmental factors and did not logically allow for the existence of any influence on the part of the individual.

Few today would advocate a purely behaviourist account of complex behaviours, and the integration of cognitive concepts (such as memories, thoughts and ideas) is now generally accepted. Indeed the cognitive–behavioural approach is now very widely adopted across branches of applied psychology and it is broadly this framework which we emphasise throughout this book as an established and effective approach to assessment and intervention.

SUMMARY

In this chapter we have outlined some of the main areas of psychology which have contributed to our understanding of criminal and delinquent behaviour.

The chapter begins with coverage of the contribution of developmental psychology. Theories of intellectual and moral development are discussed. Emphasis is given to the fact that development is lifelong and involves a complex interaction between individuals and their environment.

We go on to discuss some of the contributions of social psychology to our understanding of individual and group social behaviour. In particular, we review the contributions of research into attitudes, attributions, cognitive dissonance and group processes, looking at how these findings relate to forensic psychology.

The chapter concludes by discussing the contributions of biological psychology. This includes studies of neurological differences and the suggested role of genetic factors in criminal behaviour.

Chapter 2

The development of delinquent and criminal behaviour

INTRODUCTION

In this chapter we will look at the development of an individual and how this may impact on delinquent and criminal behaviours. It is clear that children in poor areas are more likely to be arrested and successfully prosecuted. In contrast a wide variety of antisocial behaviours may be shown by relatively privileged groups without prosecutions arising. It is possible, for example, for university students to cause serious criminal damage or commit assaults, and for this to be ascribed to 'high spirits' – an unlikely ascription for a teenager living in an economically deprived inner city area. We use the term 'delinquent' more frequently than the term 'criminal'. By delinquent we mean behaviours which are seen as socially unacceptable whether or not they result in criminal prosecutions or convictions (i.e. assaults, thefts, vandalism).

We will not cover in this chapter other developmental problems except in so far as they impinge on delinquent behaviours. So, although childhood depression, psychoses and eating disorders can all be significant aspects of development, they will not be covered. Instead we focus mainly on intellectual, social and personality development. Most of the research in this area is of North American origin. However, wherever possible we have also quoted European research and made cross-cultural comparisons. In developmental psychology the question of how universal some aspects of psychological development seen in urban–industrial cultures are, remains a key and sometimes contentious question.

INTELLECTUAL DEVELOPMENT

An individual's development is influenced from the moment of conception. Between 3 and 8 per cent of fertilised ova have genetic errors (Kopp, 1983). There are a wide range of genetically mediated disorders which will influence development. The impact of such genetic disorders varies enormously and some can be influenced and even controlled by the post-natal environment. For example, one disorder, phenylketonuria, which when untreated can lead to severe intellectual impairment, can be prevented from damaging the brain by means of a diet free of one particular chemical (phenylalanine).

A developing embryo is also vulnerable to a variety of teratogens, for example, rubella (measles), syphilis, hepatitis and human immuno-deficiency virus (HIV). In the United States 3 to 5 per cent of pregnant women are estimated to be HIV positive (Heagarty, 1991). Estimates of the rates at which mothers pass on the virus vary. One European study estimated a 13 per cent transmission rate (European collaborative study, 1991). US estimates are higher at around 30 per cent (Hutto et al., 1991). The reasons for these differences are unclear but may be linked to the quality of prenatal care available to infected mothers, and also possibly differences in sampling methods used in the research.

A wide variety of licit and illicit drugs may be taken by women during pregnancy. There are some clear conclusions from the research into the effects of these. Infants of mothers who smoke tobacco are born lighter and are twice as likely to be classified as having a low birth weight (less than 2,500 g) (Floyd et al., 1993). This seems to be due to a reduction of the placental blood supply caused by nicotine. There is also evidence of more behavioural problems in the children of mothers who smoked heavily during pregnancy (Fergusson et al., 1993).

Alcohol also has negative effects ranging from the mild to the severe. Foetal alcohol syndrome is a severe irreversible condition which pro-duces both physical changes and mental retardation. There is also some evidence that even low doses of alcohol increase the risk of damage to the foetus and that binge drinkers run a higher risk of causing damage to the foetus than regular drinkers consuming less (Olson et al., 1992). Cocaine shows a similar pattern to alcohol and children of users tend to be lighter when born. The long-term effects of cocaine are not known although it is estimated that 20–30 per cent of mothers in US inner city areas are users.

Lead is a more long-standing problem and comes now primarily from car engines. Therefore the greatest effects tend to be in urban and inner city areas where pollution is often worst. Historically, lead water pipes have also been a source of lead which is known to cause neurological damage and is associated with lowered IQ scores (Bellinger et al., 1991).

In other areas, diet, for example, the evidence is less clear. Whilst it is clear that severe malnutrition, as seen in many parts of Africa, Asia and Latin America, is very damaging indeed, chronic subnutrition, as seen in some western industrialised cultures, seems to have no direct detectable effect on foetal development (Ricciuti, 1993). In terms of the physical development of the foetus, then, the research on the mother's age is quite clear. Where prenatal care is good, then younger mothers fare better. Indeed, mothers under 18 years were less likely to produce low birth weight babies than women in their twenties (McCarthy and Hardy, 1993). Mothers over 35 years showed much higher risks of complications likely to affect foetal development.

Research has indicated a variety of gender differences in prenatal development. Within 4–8 weeks after conception male embryos begin producing testosterone. From this point girls mature slightly faster but boys are, on average, heavier and longer at birth (Tanner, 1978). Boys are also more vulnerable to a wide range of prenatal problems. Male foetuses are more likely to spontaneously abort and suffer congenital malformations and birth injuries (Zaslow and Hayes, 1986).

LOW BIRTH WEIGHT

There are two further classifications below that of low birth weight. Very low birth weight is defined as less than 1,500 g at birth (approximately 3.3 lb); and extremely low birth weight is defined as less than 1,000 g (approximately 2.2 lb). The frequency of such birth weights in western societies is declining as prenatal care improves but survival rates are increasing. In the US the risk of low birth weight is significantly increased for Afro-Americans compared to white or hispanic Americans. Mothers living in relative poverty are also significantly more likely to have low birth weight children (Reading et al., 1993).

The research suggests that children born weighing less than 1,500 g show impaired motor and intellectual development but that these children catch up quickly with those born weighing more than 1,500 g. This does not appear to be the case for those born weighing less than 1,000 g, where there is evidence of ongoing impairment and more problems at school (Collin et al., 1991).

The evidence suggests that a poor prenatal environment may make children more vulnerable to later inadequacies in their environment.

SOCIAL AND PERSONALITY DEVELOPMENT

If given the opportunity, by the time a baby is about a year old, it has normally established a clear attachment to at least one and usually more than one of its caregivers. This is displayed by means of a wide range of attachment behaviours such a smiling, crying and gazing. By the age of 2–3 years such bonds are equally strong but such behaviours are less continuously displayed. By the age of 3–4 years children still seem to have a need for someone to whom they are attached to act as a 'safe base' from which they can explore the world. However, by this stage they also seem to have developed the ability to explore progressively further away. At around the age of 4 years this attachment seems to qualitatively change, and nearly all children show significantly less distress at separation.

The role of a child's attachment to caregivers has been a focus of considerable research and debate among developmental psychologists. Early psychodynamically inspired views emphasised the importance of a single caregiver in the form of the mother (Bowlby, 1969; 1988). Whilst the descriptions of separation and separation anxiety in children produced by such research remain valid, later research has questioned the emphasis on a single caregiver. What now seems clear is that it is essential for young children to have one or more people who are a predictable and regular part of their life and to whom they can become emotionally attached. Where children lack this, they tend to have poorer long-term outcomes in terms of emotional development and also intellectual development (Rutter, 1973).

Improvements in the child's physical development also means that for the first time children are able to behave in ways which can be described as aggressive. A commonly used and helpful definition of aggression is that given by Feshbach (1970) which is that aggression is behaviour which involves the intent to injure another person or object. All children will show such behaviour at some point, although there are marked differences between individuals and also within one individual over the course of their development. Thus, some children will show very much more aggressive behaviour than others. Farrington (1993) reports that of children later exhibiting delinquent behaviour, the best predictors of this were troublesomeness at school, dishonesty and higher levels of aggressiveness than non-delinquents.

In terms of frequency, physical aggression tends to peak for the majority of children at between the ages of 2 and 4 years and declines steadily between the ages of 4 and 8 years. It tends to be replaced by verbal aggression, which becomes increasingly dominant as language skills begin to develop. The target for aggression also gradually shifts from parents towards peers. Aggressive behaviour also tends to become more severe and is more likely to be concerned with hurting others than, as at earlier ages, with obtaining something.

From an early age children in groups will form a 'pecking order' or dominance hierarchy (Strayer, 1980), and by the ages of 5 or 6, dominant children tend to be more popular with their peers (with the exception of bullies who are consistently rejected by their peers). The overall picture is that socially competent children are of middle to high levels of dominance but are positive and helpful to their peers. At this age children who are very physically aggressive tend to be rejected by their peers (Petit *et al.*, 1990).

PRO-SOCIAL BEHAVIOUR

This term is used to describe behaviours which are aimed at helping others, sharing with others or comforting those in distress. These types of behaviour can first be seen when children begin to play, usually between the ages of 2 and 3 years. One of the first pro-social behaviours seen is toy sharing. Young children often engage in this where they see another child is upset. Another is giving physical comfort by hugging or touching another child. Some 'pro-social behaviours' increase with age whilst others, such as touching, decrease. It also seems clear that individuals vary greatly in the extent to which they show such behaviours.

Research suggests that such variation is in general linked to the patterns of social interaction within the child's family. Where children show high levels of such behaviours, they tend to come from families which:

1 Show appropriate love and warmth.
2 Give clear rules and clear explanations about rules.
3 Attribute positive characteristics when children show such behaviours.
4 Encourage children to do helpful things.
5 Model thoughtful and generous behaviour.

(Bee, 1995)

Children will also begin to develop friendships from an early age. From as early as 2 years of age children show a preference for same-sex play and friendships. By around 5 years this division seems to be virtually complete (Maccoby and Jacklin, 1987). Differences in patterns of interaction between boys and girls can also be seen from this early stage. Girls tend to show a more 'cooperative' style of behaving, supporting and agreeing with each other and making suggestions. Boys in contrast tend to show a more 'domineering' style, involving contradicting, boasting and interrupting (Leaper, 1991).

It remains unclear as to precisely how such differences develop so early. There is also little research on whether these patterns are consistent across cultures. However, it has been suggested that they may be related to the child's developing sense of his or her own identity. Some theorists (e.g. Mischel, 1970) have stressed the importance of copying the behaviour of others (modelling), and finding a particular behaviour to be rewarding in some way (reinforcement). A cognitive theory to explain this process was outlined by Kohlberg (1966) who suggested that once a child develops the 'concept' that they are a boy or a girl it becomes important for them to behave in ways which enable them to be part of that group. In this model much of a child's early socialisation can be seen as being concerned with learning to behave in culturally accepted ways as a boy or girl. The child's model of gender will become more complex and more flexible with age in most cases.

ACQUIRING SELF-CONTROL

As children grow up they need to learn ways in which they can control their own behaviour rather than relying on their parents to provide such controls. Most children between the ages of 2 and 6 will gradually internalise what is and what is not acceptable and, most of the time, will control themselves accordingly. Such improvements in self-control parallel the growth in language skills already discussed.

INDIVIDUAL DIFFERENCES

It seems clear that whilst children tend to follow a similar developmental pattern within their own particular cultures, individuals within that culture will vary enormously. Such differences seem to stem from a number of sources, the two most dominant are perhaps: (1) inborn differences in temperament; and (2) styles of parenting.

Neonatal differences

More or less from birth children will show different patterns of responsiveness and temperament (see Chess and Thomas, 1984). These differences must be due to a combination of genetic differences, effects the child experienced while they were developing in the uterus and the responses and behaviours of parents to the child. Some children show patterns of behaviour which place greater demands on parents and have been described as 'difficult'. Such children tend to cry more and sleep more poorly. Such 'difficult' children are more likely to show behavioural problems later, although the vast majority do not.

Parenting

Family functioning has been conceptualised as being on four dimensions:

1 Nurturance or warmth.
2 Firmness and clarity of control.
3 Level of maturity demands.
4 Degree of communication between parent and child.

(Baumrind, 1972)

Each of these aspects of family functioning have been shown to have an influence on later behaviour.

Children from families with high levels of nurturance and warmth tend to be more securely attached to their family in the early years of life, and later show greater self-esteem, empathy and altruism towards others. They also on average have higher IQ scores and are less likely to show either delinquent or criminal behaviour later in life (Maccoby, 1980; Schaefer, 1989; Simons *et al.*, 1989). Children in otherwise economically deprived circumstances also seem to be helped where there are high levels of family nurturance and warmth. McCord (1982) found that of boys growing up in single parent families in a deprived US inner city area, those whose mothers were rated by observers as lacking warmth were three times as likely to show delinquent or criminal behaviour as the children of mothers not rated as lacking these characteristics.

Clarity of control is also highly significant. Children whose parents have clear and consistent rules are much less likely to show defiance or non-compliance with requests. Children from such families also tend to be more competent and less aggressive (Baumrind, 1972; Patterson, 1980). The best outcomes for the children seem to be linked to approaches which emphasise explaining rules, consistently enforcing them and avoiding physical punishments.

Maccoby and Martin suggest that there are four clear family types:

1 *Authoritarian.* Here demands and control are primary and families are rejecting and unresponsive.
2 *Authoritative.* Such families are demanding and controlling but also accepting and responsive to the child's other needs.
3 *Indulgent.* Such families are accepting and responsive but make few or no demands and exercise little control.

4 *Neglecting*. As the name implies such families neglect their children exercising little control and offering little acceptance or responsiveness.

(Maccoby and Martin, 1983)

The most successful approach in terms of social development in children is the second approach. The most damaging is the fourth. This tends to be confirmed by a study which found that families which show inconsistent discipline, rejection, harsh punishment and poor supervision are liable to show significantly increased levels of aggression towards others in their children (Eron *et al.*, 1991).

FAMILY STRUCTURES

Another important consideration in looking at the area of parenting is the question of family structures. The idea of the nuclear family even in western societies is increasingly inaccurate as a description of the families most children will experience. In non-western cultures extended kinship groups have traditionally been the norm; and indeed this was also the case throughout most of European history. Looking at the United States, Hofferth (1985) found that only 30 per cent of Anglo-American children would be living with both biological parents by the time they reached the age of 17 years. For Afro-American children the figure was 6 per cent. Indeed, the majority of children in the US will spend all or part of their childhood in a single-parent family. This pattern is mirrored in many western societies. However, this account masks considerable diversity in familial patterns. Indeed the term 'single parent' is often grossly misleading from a child's viewpoint where they will often be cared for by a network of kin and non-kin guardians, as well as, or instead of, the biological parents. A large number of children will also experience more than one family structure during their development.

THE IMPACT OF DISRUPTED RELATIONSHIPS

Any changes to the predictability of family structures seems to engender stress. However, this seems to be particularly problematic in cases such as divorce or separation, where the quality of family relationships is disrupted. Studies suggest that the immediate aftermath of divorce for children is often an increase in problem behaviours and a parallel decline in academic performance (Hetherington, 1989). The longer-term effects on children are less clear cut. However, what does seem clear is that the long-term negative effects in terms of delinquent or disruptive behaviours tend to be worse for boys than for girls.

This seems linked to changes in adult behaviour and parenting styles which show less evidence of authoritarian and authoritative approaches, and become more neglectful (Hetherington, 1989). This pattern seems to extend over some years and is not modified by remarriage. Such disruption of familial structures has also been shown to be correlated with later delinquent behaviour, whereas other forms of stress (such as the death of a parent) show no such relationship (Rutter, 1972). An interesting finding though is that the disruptive effects of divorce seem to be moderated where the primary caretaker (usually the mother) has another adult living with her (e.g. her mother: Dornbusch, 1985).

Interestingly this effect is not seen in families with a step-parent. Children who have step-parents show higher rates of delinquency and the parenting styles observed tend to be more authoritarian. Hetherington also found that stepfathers typically showed poor levels of rapport with their step-children and were on the whole not very involved in the process of child rearing. This was a consistent pattern over some years of study.

There is a substantial body of research on the characteristics of the families of delinquents. Such families tend to show greater extremes of rejection and indifference. Marital discord in such families also tends to be linked to conduct disorder and aggression outside the home (Loeber and Dishion, 1984).

McCord (1986) found that a lack of affection in the family between the ages of 5 and 13 years was significantly related to property crimes, whilst high levels of parental conflict and aggression were related to offences against the person. Farrington and West (1990) in a longitudinal study found a relationship between a lack of paternal involvement in a male child's interests and activities was a significant predictor of later criminal behaviour. They also found that those who were convicted of criminal acts tended to come from larger families of four or more siblings (Farrington and West, 1990). There are a variety of possible explanations for this. Farrington (1991) summarised the findings of this study in relation to delinquent behaviour. Those who became delinquent tended to come from larger families with lower incomes. They tended to have experienced unsatisfactory child-rearing practices. They also recorded lower IQ scores with one-third of the boys studied having non-verbal intelligence test scores of less than 90. They also tended to come from families with higher rates of parental criminality. Of boys who showed three or more of these risk factors, 73 per cent (46) had convictions by the age of 32 years, compared to 31 per cent of those who did not show three or more 'risk factors'.

The overall conclusion from this area of research seems to be that children approach their environment with varying levels of vulnerability. Some family environments are very protective and allow even very 'vulnerable' children to develop well. Others are unprotective or damaging, and will cause problems to all but the least 'vulnerable'. There is also some evidence that a child can act to influence its environment in ways which influence the later occurrence of delinquent behaviours (Rutter *et al.*, 1964).

In a child's interactions with others it seems that it is the process, rather than the structure, of families that is important to child development. Neglect seems to be the most damaging style of child rearing. In addition, where there is conflict and tension in interpersonal relationships (as in many divorces) the outcomes in terms of delinquent behaviour tend to be poorer for the child. This is supported by research which shows that children fare worse in terms of later disruptive and delinquent behaviour, where parental relationships have been strained or poor (i.e. divorce), but that the absence of a parent (i.e. through death) did not have this effect (Rutter, 1973).

RELATING TO PEERS

Until around the age of 12 years, one striking aspect of peer group interactions is the way boys and girls will avoid mixing wherever possible. This is even more pronounced when looking at friendships rather than just interactions, which tend to be largely single sex between the ages of 7 and 12 (Gottman, 1986). Gottman also found differences in the play of boys and girls. Boys tended to have larger friendship groups, spent more time playing outside and ranged over a larger area. Girls in contrast tended to play in smaller groups or pairs, played more indoors and covered a smaller area. Gottman termed these patterns 'extensive' and 'intensive', respectively.

It seems likely that there may be some biological basis for some of the difference seen, but socialisation is also likely to have been significant by the age of 4 years onwards. It also seems to be clear that family processes can foster high levels of aggression in children, and that the processes affect both boys and girls in similar ways. Thus, families which use authoritarian styles of punishment and use harsh and capricious punishments tend to produce higher levels of aggression in both boys and girls (Offord *et al.*, 1991).

WIDER SOCIAL FORCES

Clearly there are a multitude of social forces which will impact on children outside their families and peer groups. Many children will be born into conditions of poverty. US studies also suggest that poverty is more likely to affect ethnic minority children. Poor families tend to live in worse physical conditions. Children of poorer families tend on average to have worse health and poorer health care (Garbarino *et al.*, 1991). Such findings are not confined to North America. In most western cultures they will also have more inconsistent and poorer child care arrangements. A significant factor in many industrialised nations is endemic unemployment (See Warr, 1987). This is often compounded by very disrupted urban environments. These are characterised by severely run down housing, gang cultures, disrupted family structures and widespread drug abuse.

DEVELOPING MORAL REASONING

One area of developmental psychology that is having an increasing impact on forensic psychology is moral reasoning. Piaget (1932) was the first to give an account of this in terms of cognitive psychology. However, the work of Kohlberg (1964; 1981) has been far more influential. He suggests that there are six stages in the development of moral reasoning.

- *Stage 1: punishment and obedience.* In essence the child obeys because they will be punished when they do not.
- *Stage 2: individualism.* The child follows rules when they are in its immediate interests.
- *Stage 3: interpersonal conformity.* Moral actions become those which live up to the expectations of the family or other significant groups.
- *Stage 4: social system and conscience.* Moral actions are now those which obey existing laws and rules, except in exceptional circumstances.
- *Stage 5: utility and individual rights.* Moral actions are those which achieve the greatest good for the greatest number. Rules are now seen as changeable although some values are not.
- *Stage 6: universal ethical principles.* At this stage an individual will use self-chosen ethical principles to determine what is right.

Whilst this model does seem to have some utility, it has also been criticised. There are cultural differences in the final stage of moral reasoning reached. In complex industrialised societies, stage 5 is the optimal level for the majority. In non-urbanised cultures stage 4 is usually the optimal level reached (Snarey, 1985). In line with this critics have questioned how universally applicable the model really is.

What does seem clear is that delinquents and those convicted of criminal offences tend to use earlier stages of moral reasoning than non-delinquents (Chandler and Moran, 1990). However, this appears often to relate only to accounts of their offending, and not to other areas of their lives (Clark, 1995, personal communication). Development of moral reasoning in turn seems to parallel other aspects of intellectual development. So, as children learn more complex ways of speaking, remembering and problem solving, they also develop more complex moral reasoning (Walker, 1980). This is much of the basis of the reasoning and rehabilitation approach to offenders adopted in Canada and now the UK (Ross *et al.*, 1988).

Whilst we would not wish to question the role of intellectual and moral development in the development of delinquent behaviour, the issue is perhaps more complicated than has been suggested so far. Most critically, moral and intellectual reasoning often does not predict actual behaviour; indeed Kohlberg never suggests that this would be the case. Habit seems to be a factor in a great deal of behaviour. Also, whilst something might be morally right, it may not be seen by an individual as imperative or even important. In addition the costs to an individual of behaving in a 'moral' way seem to be relevant. Finally, there is the issue of competing social pressures. Many people will behave in ways they know to be wrong when faced with social pressures to do so (see Milgram, 1963).

ADOLESCENCE

The variations in social and personality development seen in childhood continue through adolescence. However, at this stage the number of 'problem' behaviours tends to increase. The influence of the peer group will also for most increase in relation to the influence of the family.

During adolescence the number of such antisocial behaviours tends to increase and the consequences become more serious. Accurate measures of the levels of delinquent behaviour are hard to achieve. However, in the United States around 11 per cent of 15–17-year-olds will be charged with a criminal offence (Dryfoos, 1990). European estimates tend to be of a similar magnitude (Bottomley and Pease, 1986). However, the use of official crime statistics is likely to produce a significant and highly skewed underestimate of the true levels of such behaviour. This is confirmed by self-report studies of perpetrators and victims, which show much higher levels of delinquent and criminal behaviours (Bottomley and Pease, 1986).

As for conduct disorders in childhood, delinquent behaviours are much more common in boys than in girls. The more physically violent forms of delinquency show even more pronounced differences.

Gangs and delinquent peer groups seem to have a role in promoting such behaviours. Groups of delinquents seem often to share some characteristics in common. In particular they seem less accurate in their ability to interpret the behaviour of others. They also seem to have a poorer ability to learn social rules (Schonfeld *et al.*, 1988). They are also more likely to come from families with a history of antisocial or delinquent behaviour in other family members, particularly fathers. It is unclear though to what extent these differences are effects of being part of a delinquent group, and to what extent they will lead an individual to join such groups. Bee (1995) suggests that adolescent delinquents can be divided into two main groups:

1 *Socialised subcultural delinquents.* These are individuals who mix in an antisocial subculture and behave in ways which conform to the norms of that group.
2 *Unsocialised psychopathic delinquents.* Here the term psychopathic is used in its broadest sense to refer to individuals who seem to be poorly socialised. Here delinquent behaviour is seen as independent of group norms, and such individuals seem to enjoy conflict as an end in itself.

This pattern is consistent with that found in the Isle of Wight studies in the UK (see Rutter *et al.*, 1989).

Delinquent behaviour is seen at much lower levels among girls, who are even more unlikely to be involved in violent offences. This seems to be a continuation of the fact that girls tend to be less overtly aggressive than boys at all ages. However, it is clear that girls do participate in delinquent behaviours, most commonly stealing and drug abuse. A study in New Zealand looked at delinquency in girls over time and found that the rates for such behaviours rose sharply at puberty, but only where girls attended co-educational schools. The researchers suggested that this was due to the greater number of rule-breaking models for girls to copy (i.e. delinquent boys). As is the case with boys they also found a relatively small hard core of more delinquent girls who tended to have a history of aggression during childhood (Caspi *et al.*, 1993).

So it seems that there are a very wide range of what can broadly be termed 'cultural influences' on the development of children. These include mass media forms of cultural communication such as television. Television is perhaps the most powerful means of mass communication ever devised and remains unregulated in most of the world. In countries such as the United States social violence has risen in direct proportion to the availability of television (Bee, 1995). However caution is needed in ascribing too much importance to this, and it is certainly not possible to ascribe a causal role to television in this respect. Indeed countries such as Guatemala and South Africa have lower levels of television viewing than the United States but are much more violent.

The economic climate is also of very clear importance in the development of children. The effects of poverty are clearly negative, in that poorer children experience poorer education, housing and health care. Attempts to offset these deficits by active intervention have generally failed (e.g. the Headstart programmes in the US). The only exceptions to this have been programmes which intervened with families and changed the child-rearing processes used by parents (Bee, 1995).

SUMMARY

In this chapter we have looked at development from conception to early adulthood. What seems clear from the existing research is that a multitude of influences will impinge on an individual's development, many of which will increase the risk that they will become delinquent or criminal.

There are clear differences in the types and levels of delinquent and criminal behaviours shown by boys and girls. Some of these may be linked to biological differences, others seem likely to be related to the ways boys and girls are socialised. What is clear is that boys consistently develop language-based intellectual skills later than girls. They are also consistently more aggressive and disruptive in their behaviour. At later stages boys are also much more likely to show delinquent or criminal conduct. This is particularly true where violence is involved, although it does appear that the levels of delinquent and criminal behaviour in girls is increasing, with self-reported behaviour being at much higher levels than seen in official statistics.

Another clear finding from the research is that wider social forces have a marked impact on behaviour. Not least of these influences is relative levels of poverty and deprivation. In addition, cultural values appear to be central to development although this remains a very under-researched area, with most of the existing information relating to US and European cultures. Even allowing for this proviso though, it does seem clear that most children's developmental course can be shaped in ways which increase or decrease the likelihood of later delinquent or criminal behaviours.

Chapter 3

Offender profiling

In this chapter we look at offender profiling. This is an aspect of forensic psychology which has become increasingly widely known, largely through fictionalised accounts in films and on television, as well as accounts of high-profile cases which have used this method. It is also an approach which has increasingly interested police forces and the Home Office. We begin by outlining what the term 'offender profiling' means. We then go on to look at the research and practice base for this work focusing initially on detailed studies of incarcerated offenders. We then review the analysis of crime scenes and how this is used to produce profiles. Finally, we consider the application of theories from environmental psychology to offender profiling.

Offender profiling refers to the use of information from crime scenes, and also available information on convicted offenders, to infer the likely characteristics of specific offenders (Holmes and DeBurger, 1988). Elements of this approach can be seen in the writings of many crime writers. The best-known example of such a deductive reasoning approach is probably Sherlock Holmes. Indeed, Sherlock Holmes could claim to have been among the first to use, albeit fictionally, offender profiling in the solution of crimes. However, recent interest in the application of psychological methods to the solution of crimes dates back to the 1970s and the work of the Behavioral Science Unit (BSU) of the Federal Bureau of Investigation (FBI). Prior to this, individual police departments had often asked for the views of psychiatrists and psychologists on particular crimes, with very variable results. In the United States the FBI sought to formalise this and apply what was known from the behavioural sciences through the work of their BSU at the FBI academy. This unit had the explicit role of developing a more logical and coherent approach to the links between offending and offender characteristics (Ressler *et al.*, 1980).

The process of offender profiling draws on a wide range of available information and research from the crime scene. This would include: what is done to the victim; what is taken from the crime scene; and the level and nature of the violence used. Using this information inferences can then be drawn about the likely characteristics of an offender, based on what is known about those who have committed similar offences. In common with much of psychology, this is a process of using existing knowledge to generate credible ideas or hypotheses about offenders.

The goal of offender profiling is to narrow the range of likely suspects as far as possible and so aid investigators in identifying and arresting the offender. Research in this area has largely been based on the assumption that the behaviour shown at a crime scene will reflect basic consistencies in an offender's personality and behaviour. The focus of most of the research to date has been on serial or repeat crimes. The FBI researchers defined serial homicide as three or more offences with a clear period of emotional 'cooling off' between offences. This definition served to distinguish serial offending from incidents of offending where a large number of offences are perpetrated in a short time (e.g. mass killings).

The vast majority of offender profiling research has been concerned with homicide and rape, rather than with other types of offences (see Holmes, 1990), although in recent years there has been a growing interest in the application of offender profiling to other types of offences including armed robbery, kidnapping, extortion, terrorism and burglary (Herrington, 1982; Miron and Douglas, 1979).

SEXUAL HOMICIDE RESEARCH

Nearly all of the North American research in this area has been produced by the FBI. As a federal organisation, this has led to a research focus on repeat offending which has proved difficult to solve at local or state level and/or has crossed state lines within the US. Therefore much of the research has been concerned with serial homicides (both sexually and non-sexually motivated) and serial rape offenders, although the approach is also being increasingly used in crimes such as kidnapping and extortion which frequently involve federal agencies. Even so the focus has been on what are in fact statistically rare patterns of offending, such as serial rapists, rather than statistically frequent offences, for example indecent assaults. The main approaches used have been:

1 Detailed assessment of individual offenders.
2 Analysis of crime scenes.

This in turn has led the researchers to suggest motivational models for such offending (see Burgess *et al.*, 1986).

ASSESSMENT OF INDIVIDUAL OFFENDERS

In the 1970s the FBI began a process of conducting detailed structured interviews with those serial sexual murderers who were alive, in custody and were willing or able to co-operate with the interviewers. Information from these interviews was combined with the available written records on these individuals, the aim being to develop a detailed picture of such offenders to aid future investigations.

From these interviews, thirty-six men in all, the FBI team felt able to reach some tentative conclusions about such offenders. Surprisingly perhaps, many seemed to have had a relatively advantaged start in life. Of the group 92 per cent were white and 80 per cent had average or above IQ scores. More than half came from families where both parents were present and most seemed to come from economically stable backgrounds. In these respects serial sexual murderers seem to differ markedly from the characteristics of the majority of those committing homicide of-fences. As described by Wolfgang (1958) such offenders tended to be disproportionately poor, black and from socially and economically disadvantaged backgrounds (see Chapter 6 for a fuller discussion of the characteristics of violent offenders).

In addition the FBI have also conducted studies of larger samples of those committing sexual and non-sexual homicides. These studies have generally included both serial and single homicide perpetrators.

Based on the interview data of serial sexual homicide offenders the FBI researchers suggested that many of the families of serial killers were in fact quite dysfunctional. Around 70 per cent reported, for example, a family history of alcohol abuse. In addition, over half reported a family history of psychiatric disorder, often combined with an associated history of aggression linked to the disorder. Around half the group also reported a family history of criminality.

According to those interviewed there were also problems in the nature and quality of family interaction. A high level of instability was reported and over 40 per cent reported living outside the family home before the age of 18 years. This was primarily in foster homes, state homes, detention centres or mental hospitals (Ressler *et al.*, 1993).

The majority of offenders reported an unsatisfactory relationship with their father and many seemed ambivalent about the quality of their relationship with their mothers. Many also reported parental discipline which was unfair, hostile, inconsistent and abusive.

The researchers were particularly interested in the sexual histories of these offenders. As adults nearly half the group studied reported an aversion to sex, and around 70 per cent felt themselves to be 'sexually incompetent'. A strong preference for visual sexual material was also evident for preferred sexual interests, with pornography being ranked highest.

BEHAVIOURAL INDICATORS

The FBI team felt that behaviours and experiences at various stages of life would be important indicators of later motivation to kill. They provided a detailed breakdown of what they curiously termed 'behavioural indicators'. These included behaviours such as chronic lying, compulsive masturbation and enuresis. However, they also include daydreaming, nightmares and poor body image; these might more accurately be described as cognitive rather than behavioural indicators.

Clearly there are a variety of problems with this information. For some of these behavioural indicators there are problems in achieving any consistent definition between interviewers (for example, for compulsive masturbation). Other items listed are difficult to interpret in a meaningful way. So, for example, the content of daydreams is probably important but the fact that 81 per cent of such offenders reported daydreaming tells us little of value. Even so, such findings do suggest possible avenues for further research based on more detailed assessments of offenders.

What does seem clear from these behavioural indicators is that a high proportion of these offenders performed poorly in terms of academic and work performance. Many showed poor levels of academic performance well below what might have been expected on the basis of their IQ scores. Similarly, employment records for many were unstable. Of those who had served in the armed forces (14 out of 36) 58 per cent had received dishonourable, undesirable or medical discharges. Whilst the FBI researchers do not provide information on how this compares with other groups of offenders in the US, it is perhaps significant that such a high proportion of serial killers had been trained within the armed forces. One of the serial killers interviewed by the FBI team described the onset of his deviant fantasies as changing from ones in which he was the victim, to ones in which he victimised others, as following his experiences in the Vietnam war.

It is also interesting to note that 25 out of the 36 offenders had been referred for psychiatric evaluation during childhood or adolescence. In most of these cases the response had been one of non-intervention, although in some it appeared that the offender's developing ways of thinking had been inadvertently allowed to develop. For example, Ressler *et al.* (1993) cite a case where a child's increasing interest in sadistic behaviour towards animals was thought by child guidance staff to be normal behaviour for a boy.

COGNITIVE FACTORS

Whilst this aspect of the FBI's research is in many ways even more speculative than the behavioural aspects, it does suggest some interesting ideas about the development of serial killers. As a group it seemed that these offenders were:

1 Aware of a long-standing preoccupation with and preference for a very active fantasy life.
2 Devoted to violent and sexualised thoughts and fantasies.

Based largely on ideas in cognitive psychology (e.g. Beck, 1967) it has been suggested that thinking patterns and sadistic fantasies provide the motivating drive towards sexual murder (Brittain, 1970; MacCulloch *et al.*, 1983). Whilst still largely speculative, it is argued that such offenders develop violent and sexualised fantasies early in their lives and come to prefer these fantasies to the 'real world'. However, the stresses caused by the intensity of some of these fantasies may often prepare the way for acting out such thoughts and ideas (Schlesinger and Revitch, 1980).

OFFENDING BEHAVIOURS

Moving on from the developmental cognitive and behavioural indicators, the FBI researchers suggest that the actual offence of serial murder can be broken down into distinct elements.

1 Antecedent behaviour and planning.
2 The crime scene.
3 Post-crime behaviours.

Antecedent behaviour and planning

This refers to the immediate background to the offence(s) in terms of the offender's behaviour and state of mind. The interviews conducted by the

FBI suggested a range of precipitating stresses. For this group it appeared that occurrences such as disagreements with parents or spouses could act as triggers to homicidal violence.

Immediately prior to offending a variety of emotional states were reported including:

frustration	50 per cent
hostility and anger	46 per cent
agitation	43 per cent
excitement	41 per cent
nervousness	17 per cent
depression	14 per cent
fear	10 per cent
calm	9 per cent
confusion	7 per cent.

The range of emotional states reported is clearly of interest. However, the FBI researchers appear to go beyond a reasonable interpretation of this by suggesting that these self-reports show a relative absence of 'any sense of vulnerability' so allowing the offender to interpret victim behaviour negatively (Ressler *et al.*, 1993).

They also suggest that most if not all of these offenders lack what they somewhat vaguely term an 'emotional reservoir' which would allow them to relate to, and empathise with, the vulnerability, pain and fear felt by their victims. Whilst this notion certainly has an intuitive appeal, we feel that it is fair to suggest that it is at best informed speculation.

The evidence on the planning of crimes is clearer. Half of the serial murderers studied by the FBI report pre-planning in terms of who, when and where they intended to murder. Of those who answered, 34 per cent reported being aware that their mood was in line with the offences when they planned to offend (i.e. feelings of anger or frustration). The remainder reported that the acts were spontaneous and unplanned. The FBI researchers questioned this, and they suggest that a higher proportion of such offences probably involved fantasy and planning, including some cases where the offender claimed the act was spontaneous. It is interesting to note that the FBI researchers took most of what offenders told them at face value, but decided not to accept this particular point. There are a variety of possible explanations for this. To accept that the acts of violence were spontaneous and unplanned would run counter to the model being proposed by the FBI. Also the idea that behaviour is spontaneous and unplanned is not supported by research in other areas of psychology. More prosaically the evidence in many cases did not support the idea of an unplanned attack, for example, where the victims were all of similar age, gender and appearance it seems reasonable to interpret this as a result of planning rather than chance.

Profiling of this group of offenders also suggests a range of behaviours which occurred prior to the murders and seemed to move them towards actually committing offences, rather than fantasising about them. These included the committing of burglary offences, often involving the theft of particular items such as underwear. Another factor appeared to be increased drug or alcohol abuse. This may have served to disinhibit the offender, so making it easier for them to offend.

The immediate triggers prior to a murder were defined quite broadly by the FBI to include emotional states. In at least some cases the final 'trigger' to kill the victim seems to have been the mismatch between each offender's fantasy about what they expected to happen, and the victim's actual behaviour.

The crime scene

What we have discussed so far is concerned primarily with the background to offences. However, offender profiling in practice involves taking the evidence available at a crime scene or scenes and working backwards from this to provide a profile of possible suspects. In looking at crime scenes of serial homicides the FBI uses two categories: organised and disorganised (see Holmes, 1990).

Organised offenders

The profile for such offenders suggests that:

- They tend to be high in the birth order of the family, often being the first-born.
- They are of average or above average IQ, but often are working in occupations below their abilities.
- They have histories of working in skilled occupations but their work history is uneven.
- They experience situational stressors, such as interpersonal, family or work-related difficulties prior to committing an offence.
- They tend to be socially adept and are often living with a partner.
- They may report being depressed or angry at the time of the offence.
- They are likely to have and use a car in the offence.
- They are likely to keep 'souvenirs' of the offence.
- They are likely to keep news clippings of the offence.

The crime scene of organised offenders tends to suggest some degree of order both pre- and post-offence. The crimes seem to involve a high degree of planning and systematic attempts to avoid detection. The victim is frequently a stranger and these offenders may spend a great deal of time looking for what they see as a suitable victim (i.e. one who they see as according with their fantasies about offending).

Organised offenders tend to have relatively good social skills and several developed pseudo-relationships with victims. Others started conversations or used persuasion as methods of capturing potential victims. Subsequently these offenders went on to use other means to control their victims before killing them, and these included the use of weapons as well as physical restraints. A clear example of two such offenders were the Hillside Stranglers who committed a series of sexual homicides in California.

Some of the offenders studied by the FBI reported that they killed the victims as a way to avoid detection, and that their primary motive for offending was rape.

Disorganised offenders

These offenders tended to have below average IQs and tended to be later in the birth order. Many reported harsh parental discipline during their childhood. The fathers of these individuals and the offenders themselves tended to have unstable and inconsistent work records. These offenders also tended to be much less socially competent than the organised offenders and tended to live alone or with parents, often living close to the scene of their crimes. Some were fearful of other people whilst others had developed well-defined delusional systems.

The behaviour of disorganised offenders tended to suggest impulsive behaviour whilst under stress, and the targeting of victims in close proximity to their home. Such offenders tended not to have had adult sexual relationships. Many showed high levels of ignorance about sexual matters and many seemed aversive to the idea of adult sexual relationships.

The FBI researchers suggest that the crime scenes of this group give the impression of a lack of planning, and show little evidence of attempts to avoid detection. Whilst the victims were sometimes known to the offender, the age or gender did not seem to be important in many cases. In some cases victim selection was entirely random, and the fantasy and preplanning seemed to focus on the use of violence in general, rather than focusing on fantasies about particular 'types' of victims or individuals. In other cases it appears that the homicidal violence was triggered by delusional beliefs.

These offenders tended to use a great deal more violence than was needed to kill the victim, and they tended to kill very quickly. They also tended to 'depersonalise' the victim by mutilation of parts of the body. It has been suggested that the use of very excessive force (e.g. repeated stabbing) is itself an attempt to depersonalise the victim (for example, by destruction of the victim's face). Such offenders tend to engage in only minimal interaction with their victims, mainly in the form of threats and orders. Restraints were rarely used, perhaps because the victims tended to be killed quickly.

Sexually sadistic behaviours among this group tend to be apparent postmortem. This often included evidence of urination, defecation and ejaculation over victims. Mutilations of the face, genitals and breasts occurred in many. Disembowelment, amputation and vampirism were also seen in some cases; and disorganised offenders were more likely to keep bodies or body parts as 'souvenirs' of their offending.

The crime scenes of such offenders tended to be similarly disorganised, although bodies in some cases were positioned in ways which had some meaning to the offenders. Little or no attempt was made to conceal fingerprint and footprint evidence which was frequently present at such crime scenes.

Post-crime behaviours

Among serial homicide perpetrators, a range of immediate responses to an offence were reported. These ranged from emotional relief, through to carefully planned evasion. The FBI researchers identified four patterns of post-crime behaviour of particular interest to investigating agencies.

1 *Returning to the scene of the crime.* This occurred in 27 per cent of a sample of 118 sexual murderers (both serial and single offence) (Ressler *et al.*, 1993). Of those who did this 26 per cent said it enabled them to relive their fantasy, 19 per cent said it let them check on police progress, 8 per cent did so to kill another person at the same place and 6 per cent returned to have sex with the corpse.

2 *Observing the discovery of the body.* Some of the offenders studied enjoyed the discovery of the body since they reported this allowed them to maintain their levels of excitement. Some telephoned or wrote to the police as a way to do this. Other offenders seemed to gain equal

excitement from the non-discovery of the body, since this allowed them to have a secret.

3 *Keeping 'souvenirs'.* This refers to the keeping of items connected with the offence by the offender and was reported in 27 per cent of cases. Such souvenirs seem to activate and act as a catalyst for further fantasies for offenders. These will range from items of clothing and belongings through to body parts.

4 *Participating in the investigation.* Twenty per cent of those studied participated in the investigation of their own offences. This generally involved helping the police to search for the body, or volunteering information to the police. This seemed to maintain the high level of excitement reached through their offending. A further 46 per cent followed the investigation of their crime(s) closely on television and in the press, and seemed to derive pleasure from the attention their actions had gained.

In addition, the method of killing seemed to predict some of the post-crime behaviours seen. Using a sample of 64 cases, those offenders who used a firearm only were compared with those who used only a blunt or sharp instrument to kill their victim. Those using firearms were more likely to keep a diary of their offending (56 per cent versus 26 per cent); they were more likely to keep news clippings (64 per cent versus 26 per cent) and followed their case more closely on television (82 per cent versus 50 per cent). The firearms users were also slightly more likely to confide in someone about what they had done (21 per cent versus 11 per cent).

CRIME SCENE ANALYSIS: HOW IT'S DONE

This involves practitioners in making hypothetical deductions based on:

1 The evidence available at one or more crime scenes.
2 Their knowledge about behaviour and offending in general.

The key assumption behind this approach to profiling is that thoughts, fantasies and memories (cognitive factors) drive much of the behaviour shown, and so give valuable clues about the offender. An exceptionally good fictional account of this process is given by Thomas Harris in his novel *The Red Dragon* (Harris, 1982).

The National Center for the Analysis of Violent Crime (NCAVC) of which the FBI's behavioural science unit is now a part currently divides profiling into four stages:

1 Profiling inputs.
2 Decision-process models.
3 Crime assessment.
4 Criminal profile.

These stages are followed by investigation and hopefully apprehension, which in turn feeds back into stage one.

Profiling inputs

In essence this is all the information available to a practitioner on a particular offence or group of offences. These 'inputs' would therefore include descriptions of the crime scene and areas of the crime. Descriptions of factors such as the weather and social or political climates may also be significant.

To this is added information on the victim and forensic evidence from the scene. Information on possible suspects is not included at this stage. This is done on the basis that this could distort the development of an accurate profile.

Decision-process models

This involves turning the raw information from stage one into meaningful patterns of behaviour. This is done on the basis of what is already known about particular types of offending, and in the case of homicide, NCAVC use a seven-point system to do this. This is a typology of violent crimes, and below we outline their typology for homicide offences.

Homicide type and style

Homicides are typed into categories as:

- Single homicides (one victim).
- Double homicides (two victims as one event at one location).
- Triple homicides (three victims as one event at one location).
- Mass homicide (four or more victims at one location and as part of a single event). This in turn is divided into 'classic' (i.e. non-familial) and familial mass homicides.
- Spree homicide (i.e. a series of killings without any emotional cooling-off period and at more than one site or involving more than one event). Examples of this type of offence include the Hungerford Massacre in the UK, or Charles Whitman, who killed sixteen students in Austin, Texas.

- Serial (i.e. a series of three or more separate homicide offences with an unspecified emotional cooling-off period between offences at different sites and involving separate events).

(Ressler *et al.*, 1985)

Whilst on average these groups appear to show some marked differences in characteristics they are by no means mutually exclusive. For example, Ressler *et al.* (1993) quote the example of Christopher Wilder, an Australian businessman who committed a string of carefully planned serial murders of young women in the US. When tracked down by police he went on a killing spree. This switch from serial to spree killing has been seen in other cases and it has been suggested that it may be linked to the increasing stress felt by offenders as their capture becomes likely (Douglas *et al.*, 1986).

Crime assessment

This involves attempts to reconstruct the behaviour of both the offender and the victim. Assessments are made about the classification of the crime in terms of being organised or disorganised, and also about the victim selection and offender motivations. Another consideration at this point is also whether a crime has been staged to be deliberately misleading to the investigating authorities.

The criminal profile

This is the generation of a detailed profile of the likely characteristics of the offender. Very much an art rather than a science this involves the practitioner in linking the crime analysis to the existing information on similar offenders. Such profiles in turn allow the investigating authorities to target their inquiries based on the most likely suspects in terms of demographic and background characteristics, physical characteristics and pre-offence behaviours.

VIOLENT OFFENDER CRIMINAL APPREHENSION PROGRAM (VICAP)

VICAP is a computerised information centre designed to collect, collate and analyse information on violent crimes in the US. Currently, VICAP holds information on:

1 Solved or unsolved homicides and attempted homicides where the offence has involved abduction, is apparently random or motiveless or seems to have been sexually motivated.
2 Missing persons where foul play is suspected.
3 Unidentified dead bodies where the cause of death is thought to be homicide.

The VICAP system is also planned to be extended to include rape, child sexual abuse and arson.

The purpose of VICAP was planned to be the analysis of large amounts of information about types of offences. As such VICAP can be seen as a tool to collect and analyse the types of information used by the BSU and NCAVC to develop offender profiles. As with all such computerised systems this has the advantage of allowing large amounts of information to be analysed more quickly.

ALTERNATIVE APPROACHES TO OFFENDER PROFILING

Subsequent research has drawn on the FBI and NCAVC research and in the UK this has focused on the detailed analysis of particular groups of offenders such as homicide perpetrators (Crighton, 1989; Needs, 1989) and rapists (e.g. Scully, 1990).

A very distinct development in the UK though has been the attempt to apply models and methods from environmental psychology to offender-profiling work. This research has tended to focus on more frequent offences such as burglary, although some work has also concerned rapists.

Canter *et al.* (1990) suggest six main principles based on such environmental research.

1 *Distance decay.* Essentially this is the idea that offenders will commit fewer offences as the distance from their home increases. The vast majority of this research is based on methodologically flawed studies of domestic burglaries (e.g. Stone, 1989). Canter *et al.* carried out a similar analysis for a sample of 15 serial rapists and found a similar effect for these offenders.
2 *Familiarity.* This refers to the idea that individuals will tend to offend in areas that they are familiar with.
3 *Criminal range.* This is the idea that offenders will vary in terms of the distances they will range over to offend. This in turn seems to be linked to several other factors such as access to transport, the degree

of pre-planning of the offence and the extent to which the offender travels in other contexts.

4 *Safety zone.* This refers to the tendency for offenders not to commit offences in very close proximity to their homes (Turner 1969). Phillips (1980) suggests that one very obvious explanation of this might simply be ease of recognition.

5 *Mental buffers.* This is the notion that an individual's psychological representation of the world is not exactly the same as geographical reality. In particular, such mental representations tend to contain mental barriers, such as the divisions between particular areas. In addition, an offender's ideas about distances may have little bearing to real distances (Baker and Donnelly, 1986).

6 *Temporal changes.* This is the suggestion that offenders will range further away from home as their offending progresses. However, there is no consistent evidence to support this to date.

7 *Differences between types of crime.* Brantingham and Brantingham (1981) suggested that 'emotionally' motivated crimes (e.g. sexual or violent crimes) would show lower levels of search or planning than instrumental crimes such as burglary.

8 *The circle hypothesis.* This proposes that offending will occur within a relatively fixed distance of the offender's home, which will act as a central focus (Canter *et al.*, 1990).

CRITICISMS OF OFFENDER PROFILING

The clearest criticism of the FBI and NCAVC studies is the very heavy reliance on offenders' self-reports of:

1 Their own backgrounds.
2 Their offending behaviour.
3 Their victim's behaviour.

More recent research, however, has attempted to corroborate offenders' accounts. Some aspects of an offender's behaviour are also only available through self-report (e.g. an offender's fantasies). However, it is clear from many studies that offenders may systematically distort aspects of their background and behaviour to justify their offending (see Murphy, 1990). Curiously the FBI researchers seem to have taken much of the self-report information gleaned at face value, whilst drawing little from the experience and research of other practitioners working with offenders.

It is also of concern that most of the US-based research has not included a comparison of the factors identified in profiling work with a control group of people with similar backgrounds who have not offended, or have offended in different ways. So, for example, they emphasise the fact that 81 per cent of sexual homicide offenders in their studies report daydreaming. This is a methodological weakness of such research because they have not compared this rate (81 per cent) to the level found in other types of offenders or non-offenders.

Overall, much of the US research is descriptive rather than analytic. So the fact that 28 per cent of these offenders reported a history of cruelty to animals is difficult to interpret without knowing what the levels of such behaviours are in the general population and also in other criminal groups. In this respect the researchers missed an opportunity to outline the distinctive characteristics of such offenders (see Capsan, 1996; Olson, 1996).

CRIME SCENE ANALYSIS AND PROFILING

The distinction between organised and disorganised offenders has an intuitive appeal. It also appears to have utility to those investigating crimes. However, there is little empirical evidence to support the clear separation of these groups. Thus, the use of drugs or alcohol is likely to overlap both groups. The distinction seems to imply a group of relatively intelligent and socially skilled offenders, who use these skills to entrap victims, against a group of less intelligent, socially unskilled offenders, who rely on the use of physical force alone. Whilst this distinction is claimed to be useful in investigations of crime, we would suggest that this is an area which would benefit from considerable further research, for example, research drawing on the wider range of knowledge of practitioners working with such offenders.

ENVIRONMENTAL PSYCHOLOGY APPROACHES

This approach to offender profiling has tended to focus on more frequent crimes such as domestic burglaries, although some studies have looked at rape offenders. The results of this approach will, for many, be disappointing in terms of yielding new or valuable insights into offenders. For example, the idea that most burglaries are committed within easy range of an offender's home but not in the immediate environment is perhaps unsurprising. It seems unlikely to add anything to existing police strategies for the detection of such crimes.

In other respects the approach uses a crass and simplistic level of analysis upon which to base distinctions between offenders. Research in this area often seems to have ignored other research into the behaviour of offenders. For example, the idea that 'emotional' offenders will show less evidence of planning than 'instrumental' offenders suggests a worryingly simplistic level of analysis. The FBI and NCAVC research suggests that serial homicide and rape offenders will often spend a great deal of time planning and fantasising about their offences. This is similarly true of many sexual offenders against both adults and children. In contrast, many acquisitive offences such as robbery or burglary may often show little or no evidence of planning, whilst some acquisitive offenders (e.g. armed robbers) will tend to show a great deal of systematic planning in their crimes.

SUMMARY

In this chapter we have reviewed research into offender profiling. The vast majority of this research has been conducted in North America. Initial studies were concerned to produce detailed analyses of the relatively small numbers of offenders who had committed sexual and non-sexual serial homicides. These analyses included background characteristics, behaviour prior to offending, during offending and post-offence. Later work has extended to include studies of serial rapists, arsonists, terrorists, extortionists and burglars.

The main application of offender profiling has been 'crime scene analysis'. Here, particular aspects of a crime scene are used to determine whether an offender is 'organised' or 'disorganised' in their offending. This distinction is suggested to be of value in predicting characteristics of the perpetrator. We have outlined how this is done.

In the UK there has been a considerable amount of research using similar approaches to those of the FBI and National Center for the Analysis of Violent Crime (NCAVC) in the USA. A distinctive approach has also developed drawing on environmental psychology and environmental criminology. The results of this approach have been generally quite prosaic and disappointing in terms of how far they have increased understanding of criminal behaviour, or improved the detection of crime.

Part II

Assessing risk

Chapter 4

Risk assessment

INTRODUCTION

Practitioners will sometimes complain that we can never be certain about our decisions associated with risk assessment. Their argument is that there will always be a chance that we will be wrong, resulting in sometimes tragic consequences for clients and potentially damaging consequences for professionals. Such concerns may sometimes result in the forensic field in practitioners adopting defensive professional practices (Harrison, 1995). One fundamental difficulty that such professional assertions reflect is the somewhat confused and varied usage of the term 'risk'.

In this chapter we explore and examine what the term 'risk assessment' encompasses. In our examination of the term we draw from other fields where problems of risk assessment have been ably grappled with. Our primary focus is to give the practitioner a working definition of risk assessment linked to an explicit framework to help structure effective decision making. The framework for risk assessment that we describe may be legitimately applied across a range of areas, both within and outside of the forensic field.

Problems of risk assessment are by no means exclusive to the forensic field. Issues of risk assessment concern a broad range of disciplines, including economics (e.g. Hey, 1979), engineering (e.g. Cooper and Chapman, 1987), sociology (e.g. Luhmann, 1993) and anthropology (e.g. Douglas, 1992). The broad range of disciplines concerned with issues of risk assessment may well contribute to the lack of an agreed definition of precisely what it involves. However, the range of perspectives given across different disciplines provides us with a rich vein of ideas and practices which have concrete and helpful applications for practitioners in the forensic field.

A pervasive theme and tension across a number of disciplines addressing issues of risk assessment is the extent to which 'scientific knowledge' may inform and improve our risk assessment practices. Indeed, some authors in the area have suggested that what we need is a conceptual framework into which all the scientific and social aspects of risks can be fitted (Council for Science and Society, 1977). Our aims for this chapter are far more modest. From our assessment of this area it seems to us that although certain aspects of the risk assessment process may be trans-scientific, i.e. they may require solutions beyond the practical application of a scientific method, many aspects of the risk assessment process do benefit from such an approach. More precisely, we may utilise a scientific approach in identifying the probabilities of occurrences of target behaviours and the monitoring of future behaviour. We would distinguish these procedures and practices from the process of decision making about what should be done in the light of target behaviours being identified and probabilities of their occurrence being estimated. Notions of the acceptability or otherwise of taking particular decisions based on a rigorous risk assessment procedure have nothing to do with 'scientific method': such decisions are rooted in moral and ethical considerations about individual and collective rights and responsibilities.

One particularly misleading yet pervasive notion across disciplines in addressing issues of risk assessment is the notion that if something goes wrong (e.g. an aeroplane crashes despite all relevant safety checks and procedures being implemented) then the initial risk assessment decision was wrong. In this example the risk assessment decision was, presumably, that the plane was safe to fly. We believe the logic of the argument that the decision was 'wrong' to be fundamentally flawed. The correctness of a risk assessment decision is based upon a combination of the methodology used to inform the risk assessment process and the ethical basis of the decision making taking account of:

1 An estimate of the consequences of a target event occurring.
2 An estimate of the probability of the target event's occurrence.

Such muddled thinking is in part based upon a basic misunderstanding of the nature of risk assessment. Risk is the antithesis of certainty. We live in a predominantly uncertain world. We will never be able to demonstrate that our risk assessments will always be right in the sense of achieving their desired outcome. Thus, a plane may crash despite all reasonable steps being taken to ensure the safety of its passengers. It does not follow therefore that we should not fly! Although, of course, we are free to make such a decision based on an understanding of the probability of occurrence of the crash and the consequences of it.

DEFINITIONAL ISSUES

It is perhaps helpful at this stage in our discussion to deal further with some definitional issues. The literature is riddled with muddled definitions. The term 'risk' is sometimes used to refer to an outcome (e.g. someone committing suicide). It is sometimes used as a statement of probability. More often, it is used as a combination of both probability and outcome. Needless to say this often leads to confusion. Notions of 'risk' are often associated with negative consequences. We believe that in forensic practice 'risk' is most helpfully understood as a statement of probability in relation to a specified target behaviour. The target behaviour may be 'positive' or 'negative'. Our definition of risk assessment is: *a combination of an estimate of the probability of a target behaviour occurring with a consideration of the consequences of such occurrences.* This definition makes no implicit assumptions about the desirability or otherwise of target behaviours. The term 'target behaviours' may be used to cover virtually any behavioural category, e.g. sex offending, violence or suicide.

We set out a framework for practitioners which may function as an *aide mémoire* when doing risk assessments (see Figure 4.1). It also puts our definition in the context of the risk assessment process.

RISK ASSESSMENT: HOW TO DO IT

The first thing to do is to specify clearly what the target behaviour is that we are concerned with. For example, we may be concerned that an adult offender will sexually assault a young child. We view this as stage 1 of the risk assessment process.

Next, we need to specify what it is that makes us think that the adult in question will sexually assault a young child. Perhaps he has previously offended against children. In our framework, we move to the beginning of stage 2 of the risk assessment process. We examine the knowledge base. In this example we would look at what is known about sexual offending, specifically against children. We may, for example, look at actuarial data, i.e. statistical data on reoffending rates. It is important that when looking at such data, if at all possible, to check that the sample it is based upon matches some basic characteristics of our individual client. For example, rape statistics are often based on samples of those have been sentenced to prison. Such samples will be largely working class. Middle-class rapists are considerably less likely to be taken to court or to be found guilty of rape. Another key factor of such data is the time

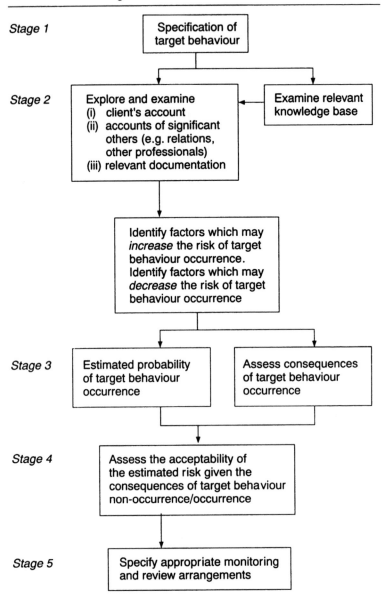

Figure 4.1 A practitioner's framework for risk assessment

frame which is used between the start point (often release from custody) of the data collection to the termination of data collection. Studies giving statistical data on reoffending for sex offenders are often based on data collected over a 2-year follow-up period. On occasion, the data are collected for a 5-year period. Recorded reoffending rates will be quite different under the 2-year and 5-year conditions. The offender will have had more than twice the opportunity to offend over the 5-year period compared with the 2-year follow-up period. Also, such statistical studies are generally based upon reconvictions rather than reoffending. Other types of studies in the general area of sex offending tend to indicate that relying on such data would be to underestimate seriously the chances of reoffending.

So when looking at statistical data it is important to try to ensure that the characteristics of the population used are similar to your client's. Also, to improve the accuracy of risk assessments it is important to note the temporal parameters used in studies and how they match the time frame you will use. It is often good practice to use the same time frame for risk assessment as those in the studies alluded to, e.g. 2 years.

In our examination of the general knowledge base in the area, we would be looking at the characteristics of offenders who exhibit the target behaviour we have specified (i.e. to sexually assault a young child). Here, a knowledge of the characteristic cognitive distortions and behavioural patterns of such offenders will be useful (for a fuller discussion of this area see Chapter 10). A theme throughout our examination of the current knowledge base is that we constantly attempt to match the information from the literature with our information about our client.

When examining the individual case we have found an approach sometimes referred to as functional analysis of behaviour to be useful (for a more detailed discussion of this approach see, for example, Owens and Ashcroft, 1982). A feature of this approach is to look at the functions of particular behavioural patterns for the offender. A number of different acronyms may be used to assist this assessment process. For example, BARE-PC, which stands for behaviour, attitudes, relationships, emotions, personality and cognitions. The essence of an assessment of an individual case such as the one we describe is to get a good understanding of the offender's world. In other words, we need to understand how the offender views himself in relation to others. We would not wish to be overly prescriptive about which approach to take to ascertain the necessary understanding of the offender's world. One may draw from many different approaches, e.g. personal construct theory (PCT) (Kelly, 1955). One helpful application derived from PCT in the forensic field has been Needs' (1988, 1995) WOMBAT. WOMBAT stands for 'Way Of Me Behaving And Thinking'. This integrative unit is used to explore and examine relevant aspects of behaviour, beliefs, self-statements, ways of coping and situational contexts with the client. We have found it to be a useful exploratory tool. Cognitive–behavioural approaches may also be helpfully applied. We would draw primarily from cognitive–behavioural approaches in our work with offenders. Whichever approach is used it is essential that the practitioner aims at getting as full an understanding as possible of how an offender views himself in relation to others as a critical component of any risk assessment process.

There are also psychometric tests which may be used to aid our assessments. These can be particularly useful in helping us structure the particular aspects of the offender's profile which may be of concern to us. Some psychometric tests are also helpful as tools to help measure the efficacy of our subsequent interventions aimed at reducing the risk of specific reoffending.

Concurrent to getting the offender's account of himself and events, it is important to examine thoroughly documentation and records germane to the case. Also, it may be helpful to speak to significant others in the offender's life, e.g. his wife. Such information is important, especially in seeking corroborative accounts of critical events.

The findings of the inquiry into the widely publicised case of Christopher Clunis bear testimony to the importance of seeking corroborative accounts of events, from sources other than the individual client in making our assessments. This was not something done by the psychiatrists involved in this case (Lingham, 1995). Clinical experience in the forensic field thus provides us with a salutary reminder of the need to seek corroborative evidence of our client's account of events.

In our case example we have clearly specified the target behaviour we are concerned with – 'the risk of sexually assaulting a young child' – and we have looked at how we might go about examining both the general area of sexual offending and an understanding of the individual offender.

Once we have completed our examination of both the knowledge base in the relevant area and have carefully assessed the individual case before us, we may focus upon the central business of the identification of factors which may *increase* the risk of the target behaviour occurring. We also need to identify the factors which may *decrease* the risk of the target behaviour occurring (see Figure 4.1, stage 2).

Often, we suspect, a disproportionately large amount of time and effort is focused upon the factors which would *increase* the risk of reoffending. However, we would argue that factors which would *decrease,* in our case illustration, the risk of sexual assault against a child, are equally important to consider. Both sets of factors are very important and absolutely central to the risk assessment process.

The term 'factors' is a very general one and may be used at a number of levels. Generally, we may look at a combination of offenders' motivations, strategies and skills for offending and for not reoffending.

Let us suppose that the offender in our case example reports being motivated to change his behaviour. From our earlier examination of his individual case we would have an understanding of his pattern of offending, his personality and his behavioural propensities. It is incumbent upon the practitioner to share his or her concerns with the offender about the latter's pattern of offending. Strategies for behavioural change are largely based upon the notion that the offender has insight into his offending behaviour, and wishes to change it.

In looking at the pattern of offending, personality and behavioural propensities of the offender in the context of their social situation we would attempt to derive the key factors which would impact on the risk of reoffending. One behavioural factor which may increase the risk of reoffending might be the offender planning to put himself in situations which would give him greater access to potential victims. One cognitive factor which may increase the risk of reoffending might be an increasing preoccupation with sexual activity against children. Conversely, decreases in these two factors may decrease the risk of reoffending. However, it is not simply a case of looking at the converse of what would increase the risk of reoffending to ascertain a full picture of what may contribute to reducing the risk of reoffending. A number of what may be termed 'protective factors' are also important. For example, in our case illustration it may be that the offender being involved in an intimate adult relationship (free from ulterior motives such as access to children) may serve as a protective factor in reducing his risk of reoffending. We would stress that this is very much an example and it is essential that the practitioners are guided by their earlier assessment of the case in deriving such 'protective factors'. One helpful heuristic to do this can be to examine closely times in the offender's life when he has not been offending to try to tease out any environmental differences compared to times when he has been offending.

From the earlier assessment of the offender, the practitioner will have a good idea of the offender's strengths and deficits in social skills. A number of these skills may directly impact upon the risk of reoffending. For example, our offender may not have the skills to initiate adult sexual contacts. Whilst such skills deficits remain, their absence may serve to increase the risk of reoffending.

In sum, the factors which may increase the risk of reoffending and the factors which may decrease the risk of reoffending may be derived from the earlier assessment, focusing upon the motivation, strategies and skills of the offender in his social context.

From stage 2 of the assessment process (see Figure 4.1) we should be in a position to draw together the two critical features of any risk assessment, namely:

1 An estimate of the probability of the target behaviour occurring.
2 An estimate of the consequences of the target behaviour occurring.

These two features constitute stage 3 of the assessment process. Essentially this is a product of the informed analysis from stage 2. Thus, we can see how stages 1 to 3 may be completed by the systematic analysis of relevant data in relation to the risk assessment process. Stage 4 involves a very different level of analysis associated with moral notions of the acceptability of the estimated risk of target behaviours occurring or not occurring.

So, stage 4 of the assessment process involves the decision-making process about the *acceptability* of the estimated risk of the target behaviour occurring. Such judgements will be very much informed by personal, professional and political considerations. Such decision making is rooted in the premise that we need to consider the rights of all interested parties in our deliberations.

Stage 5 of the risk assessment process involves the monitoring of the client. 'Risk' as a concept is not static, it is dynamic. Indeed, it is worth noting that actuarial (or statistical) information on the risk of reoffending for general offence categories are essentially static models. Offenders change, both in terms of themselves and their circumstances. It is imperative that risk factors are closely and systematically monitored. To revisit our earlier analogy of the aeroplane, monitoring involves routine safety checks. These would be regularly undertaken and documented. It seems to us to be foolhardy simply to identify 'risk factors' and not implement monitoring and review procedures in the forensic field. Monitoring also serves to further inform and perhaps call in to question our initial assessment of the offender in terms of patterns of offending.

A theme throughout the framework is the need to be explicit about the evidence we use and judgements we make in our assessments of the level of risk of a specific target behaviour (not) occurring and in estimating its consequences for each interested party.

WRITING RISK ASSESSMENT REPORTS

There are a number of rules of thumb which apply when writing most reports. An awareness of the purpose of the particular report is the essential starting point for report writing. Next, one may consider the needs and levels of understanding of the intended audience of the report. These two conditions help inform the practitioner about the most appropriate structure for the report.

Numerous texts are available on how to improve one's writing skills and style. It can also be a helpful exercise to read through the reports of experienced and able practitioners in the field. It is generally useful to get another practitioner to read through your reports to help you to identify the strengths and weaknesses.

Open reporting

Increasingly, and quite rightly, open reporting is becoming commonplace in the forensic field. This serves to increase accountability among practitioners. In practical terms it is thus more important than ever that practitioners write clear, fair and accurate reports when required. In the forensic field, this may give rise to some tensions, especially when there are competing needs or views between various interested parties affected by the report writing process. The report needs to be written in such a way that it can be justified to each party in terms of its accuracy, fairness and clarity.

Useful pointers for writing risk assessment reports

Table 4.1 is a checklist for practitioners writing risk assessment reports. It begins by mentioning the need to specify clearly the target behaviours that there is a risk of happening. This is important because it gives the reader a clear focus. Using multiple sources during the risk assessment process is especially important, partly because it is important that we learn from the outcomes of enquiries into when things have gone wrong in practitioner's assessments – seeking corroborative accounts of events from multiple sources is one such lesson. It is imperative that evidence for assertions made in reports is made explicit. This has a particularly important effect on the perceived fairness of reports for report readers. It also helps the writer to develop further the logic of the report to include a list of factors which may *increase* (or often crucially *decrease*) the risk of the target behaviour occurring.

Table 4.1 Checklist for writing risk assessment reports

1 Clearly specify target behaviour.
2 Use multiple sources in an attempt to corroborate accounts.
3 Be explicit about what evidence you are drawing from in making your risk assessments.
4 Estimate the level of risk present and what it is likely to be under specific conditions within a given time frame, e.g. 2 years.
5 List factors (e.g. those factors which may increase the risk of target behaviour occurrence and those factors which may decrease the risk of target behaviour occurrence) which require further monitoring.
6 Do *not* use the term risk to mean different things within the same report.
7 Assume that risk may generally be most helpfully construed as a continuous rather than dichotomous variable.

What not to do

Because the term 'risk' is used in so many different ways this is often reflected in report writing. Perhaps one of the most common and serious errors in the writing of risk assessment reports is to make statements which are based on the assumption that risk may be usefully construed as a dichotomous rather than a continuous variable. A continuous variable may have a broad range of possible values on a continuum. A dichotomous variable may be in one of two categories. Viewing risk as a dichotomous variable involves the assumption that 'risk' is either present, or it is not. We believe this to be a potentially very dangerous assumption. Viewing 'risk' as a continuous variable involves the assumption that 'risk' exists across a broad range of levels for any target behaviour. Such a conceptualisation affords us a more complex and sound basis on which to conduct our risk assessments.

Using our earlier case example, if we were to use a framework of risk assessment based on the assumption of risk being a dichotomous variable, we may make the assumption that our sex offender presented 'no risk'. Such an assessment would be entirely at odds with what we know about sex offenders. It may also preclude the opportunity to monitor the behaviour of the offender carefully and regularly. Despite this, sadly, some report writers continue to use such terms. Still using the 'dichotomous variable' framework, if we were to conclude that the offender was 'a risk' we would limit our opportunities to demonstrate the efficacy of future treatment interventions. For example, we may initially estimate that an offender has a high risk of reoffending. After treatment we may estimate that he has a lower risk of reoffending. Using a solely dichotomous variable framework, our 'before' and 'after' measure of treatment efficacy would indicate 'a risk' before and 'a risk' after. A continuous variable structure is more flexible, realistic and helpful for all parties concerned, at each level of the risk assessment process.

PERCEPTUAL PREJUDICES IN MAKING RISK ASSESSMENTS

Perception involves the active and passive processes of the interpretation of information. Prejudice involves judgements and opinions formed without a due examination of relevant information (i.e. making assumptions).

We have already seen how the risk assessment process necessarily includes the use of subjective judgements. Our perceptions and prejudices are likely to play a significant role in informing such subjective judgements. Indeed, there is good evidence that our judgements may be very resilient to accepting alternative evidence, which may run contrary to our existing views (Nisbett *et al.*, 1982).

Clearly, understanding our perceptual prejudices is important in developing our work in making effective decisions about risk assessment. Researchers have identified a number of 'perceptual biases which characterise important aspects of our decision making associated with predicting the probability of specified events occurring. In an influential account, Tversky and Kahneman contended that:

> people rely on a limited number of heuristic principles which reduce the complex tasks of assessing probabilities and predicting values to simpler judgemental operations. In general these heuristics are quite useful, but sometimes they lead to severe and systematic errors.
>
> (Tversky and Kahneman, 1974)

As Tversky and Kahneman point out, our 'heuristics' or short-hand perceptual rules for informing our decision making are often helpful in everyday life, but crucially contain systematic biases which may have detrimental effects on our decisions. They describe three such heuristics which they call representativeness, availability and adjustment and anchoring.

Representativeness

This refers to a group of systematic heuristic biases which are used in decision making. People tend to estimate probabilities of events occurring partly based on a notion of 'representativeness' rather than other factors which may be important. For example, in child protection work, if a practitioner is presented with two sets of case notes describing the home environments of two children, one from a middle-class background and one from a working-class background, the latter may more readily 'match' their notion of an environment where criminal activity would be more likely. Thus, they would be more likely, if asked, to assign a higher probability of the individual child becoming involved in crime. Such a heuristic may sometimes have its uses. However the fundamental problem with it here is in its application to individual cases in the light of the clear limitations of the data set on which such judgements are based. A consideration of the base rates of specified criminal activities would surely be a helpful piece of information in helping inform such decision making. However, such consideration may sometimes be overridden by the representativeness heuristic. In short then, the mistake the practitioner is making is matching the notion of 'environment' and 'criminal activity' without due consideration of other factors (e.g. base rates).

Perhaps most worryingly, people often report a high degree of confidence in many of the predictions they make even when they are manifestly inaccurate. This is sometimes referred to as the 'illusion of validity'. For example, psychological research clearly shows the severe limitations of selection interviews as a method for selecting candidates for jobs (Woodruffe, 1990). However, employers still often use this method rather uncritically.

Perhaps one of the most important applications of the representativeness heuristic in the forensic field may be misconceptions associated with (statistical) regression to the mean. We use the term 'statistical regression' here to refer to the phenomenon whereby extreme events are most liable to be followed by less extreme events. For example, we have seen that a very important aspect of the risk assessment process is the monitoring of factors which may increase and decrease the risk of target behaviour occurrence. A client may exhibit behaviour which leads the practitioner, on one occasion, to record significant progress – either because of a decrease in some behaviours or an increase in others. The chances are that the following week there will be a (at least slight) deterioration in behaviour from the immediately preceding 'highpoint' of adaptive behaviour. This does not necessarily mean that overall there has not been progress.

Availability

The availability heuristic refers to the notion that the retrieval of relevant factors from our limited memories is important in informing our estimates of the risk of target behaviour occurrences. For example, the Bolger case in Liverpool may have served to increase practitioners' concerns about children as both offenders and victims. Prior to the media attention attracted to the case it was less likely that such concerns would be retrieved from memory and thereby influence practitioners' decision making for their risk assessments. Familiarity and salience are important factors, in affecting the 'availability heuristic'.

One problem, especially in the forensic field, is that *the act of contemplating* the possibility of someone committing an offence (e.g. a homicide) may increase our perceptions of the level of risk involved. Indeed, rare causes of death tend to be overestimated (e.g. homicide) and common causes underestimated (e.g. heart disease).

Adjustment and anchoring

These refer to the phenomena whereby people make estimates (e.g. the risk of x events occurring) by starting from an initial value that is adjusted for their final risk assessment. This is the case whether or not the 'initial value' is based on an opinion or statistical information, i.e. actuarial data. In the best-case scenario, where the initial value is based on relevant actuarial data, this may be helpful initially. However, just as a number of actuarial models of reoffending are static, so may be our perceptual processes in evaluating change; for example, if a prisoner is imprisoned for a serious sexual offence after serving, say, 10 years and after undertaking treatment work their risk of reoffending may have apparently been reduced. The extent of this reduction is likely to be judged in relation to the level of offending initially apparent. This bias may reduce the accuracy of such estimates.

PERCEPTUAL PREJUDICES: WHAT CAN WE DO TO ALLEVIATE THEIR NEGATIVE EFFECTS?

We have seen how perception is important in risk assessment work (e.g. Slovic *et al.*, 1976). Thus understanding such perceptions is clearly crucial to aid effective decision making. Media representations of violent crime may serve to increase our estimates of the risk of it occurring to us or others. Indeed, reports of the public perceptions of rates of violent crime tend to overestimate dramatically the official rates. The fear of certain crimes may also effect our decision making.

The key point for practitioners must surely be to have an awareness of the potency of such perceptions and how they may impact on decision making for both practitioners and clients. We are all limited by only having a very narrow range of experiences to draw upon to help us with our decision making about a broad range of events. We have seen how it is important to draw upon actuarial data in our estimates of risk and to examine critically our perceptual prejudices.

We would emphasise that in the forensic field there is a need for such an awareness to apply to both clients and practitioners. This is especially so when we are trying to enable clients to reduce their risk of reoffending; this requires a high level of insight into the false confidence we may have about a number of our judgements related to planned strategies for reducing the risk of reoffending.

SUMMARY

In summary we have seen how it is important to use the term risk as a statement of probability about the predicted occurrence or non-occurrence of a clearly specified target behaviour. We have outlined a framework (see Figure 4.1, p. 56) to help us enable forensic practitioners to structure the process of their risk assessment work clearly. The framework may be applied to a wide range of behaviours.

Our framework has five stages:

1 The specification of the target behaviour.
2 An exploration and examination of the knowledge base in the area, linked to the elicitation of a detailed account of events from the client, significant others and the relevant documentation. This is done with a view to identifying and making explicit factors which may increase the risk of target behaviour occurrence and factors which may decrease the risk of target behaviour occurrence.
3 An estimation of the probability of target behaviour occurrence in conjunction with an assessment of its consequences.
4 An assessment of the acceptability of the estimated risk, given the consequences of the target behaviours' (non-) occurrence.
5 The specification of appropriate monitoring and review arrangements.

The utility of using the term risk as a statement of probability and therefore as a continuous variable is emphasised throughout our discussion of risk assessment. This should be reflected in report writing when making risk assessments. In Table 4.1 (p. 62) we give a brief checklist for risk assessment reports. The importance of our perceptual prejudices in our decision making is highlighted in terms of its significance in possibly affecting our judgements in relation to risk assessments. The perceptual biases of representativeness, availability and adjustment and anchoring are briefly outlined, illustrating their possibly problematic application in the risk assessment process.

Chapter 5

Risk assessment of suicide

This chapter provides the reader with an example of the application of the risk assessment model proposed in Chapter 4 of this handbook. We attempt to give the reader some general information in the area of suicide and factors which appear to be associated with its occurrence and effective management.

There are a number of definitional problems associated with examining suicide. There are a range of philosophical difficulties (see, for example, Anderberg, 1989) in defining the precise nature of suicide. These difficulties tend to be associated with such issues as intentionality and motives and knowledge. Sociologists have pointed to the importance of the social construction of official suicide figures, particularly in relation to possible distortions at coroner's courts. Indeed whether or not a self-inflicted death is recorded as a suicide is a matter of judgement for coroners. Other judgements open to them in cases of self-inflicted deaths are: death by misadventure; an open verdict; or accidental death. Notwithstanding the above definitional problems, we feel that it is important for our purposes to operationalise our use of the term 'suicide'. Our definition of suicide is *'the act of taking one's own life'*. In terms of our framework for risk assessment this definition constitutes the target behaviour for our risk assessment.

SUICIDE: AN OVERVIEW

Research information on suicide may be broken down broadly into two categories of studies: the nomothetic and the idiographic. Nomothetic studies are those studies which are characterised by demographic and statistical information. Idiographic studies have as their focus the individual and they are characterised by, for example, individual case studies. Below we draw from both types of study in order to give the reader an awareness of the range of work in this field. Each of these respective levels of description and analysis may be usefully incorporated in forensic practice. We will outline how such knowledge may be applied after we have given an overview of suicide.

Suicide rates

Estimates of the rates of suicide in different countries vary considerably. Comparative research suggests that the rates of suicide are recorded at between 3 to 45 persons a year per 100,000 of population (Diekstra and Hawton, 1987). Historically, those aged over 65 have tended to be overrepresented in the statistics. For example, in the US white men aged over 50 represent 10 per cent of the population and account for 28 per cent of the deaths by suicide (Getz *et al.*, 1987). However, there appears to be a general trend of increasing suicide rates among the 15–24-year-old group. The rate in the US in 1955 was 6 per 100,000; by 1985 this had more than tripled to 20 per 100,000. Each year over 30,000 individuals in the US take their own lives by suicide (National Center for Health Studies, 1992). For the 15–29 age group in the European Community, suicide is the third most common cause of death after road accidents and cancer. In recent years there has been a significant growth in the number of young people committing suicide both in the USA and Europe. This is also the case among women. At a general level it is worth being mindful of the fact that high-risk populations change over time, e.g. we have seen that over the last 30 years the risk of suicide among younger age groups has appreciably increased (Morgan and Owen, 1990).

Rates of suicide in prisons in England and Wales have risen dramatically in the 1980s and early 1990s, accounting for 387 deaths in custody over a 10-year period from 1984 to 1994. In 1994 the rate of suicides in prison was the highest ever recorded accounting for sixty self-inflicted deaths. Presumably this is, in part, a reflection of the trend of younger age groups being overrepresented in recorded suicide rates generally.

The social context of suicide

Not only may we distinguish between different age groups in terms of prevalence for suicide, we may also look at social contexts which play a role in contributing to differential suicide rates.

Diekstra and Hawton (1987: 1) give a picture, drawing from a broad range of research studies, of the social circumstances of those more prone to suicide. Those especially at risk are: 'youngsters from disrupted families and from families with a history of suicide, drug and alcohol addiction, those who have failed at school, the unemployed, and those suffering from depression'. This shows that some of the social conditions associated with suicide parallels those of many offenders. Indeed, such descriptions bear a remarkable resemblance to lists generated from prospective longitudinal studies of the social factors of those involved in crime (e.g. Farrington, 1993).

Economic deprivation is associated with poor physical and mental health. Since 1979, in the UK, the rich have got richer and the poor poorer (Townsend, 1993). The risk of attempted suicide rapidly increases with the length of time unemployed. For example, those unemployed for less than 6 months have six times the risk of attempting suicide than their employed counterparts. However, those unemployed for over 12 months have nineteen times the risk of attempting suicide (Platt and Kreitman, 1984). The unemployed are significantly overrepresented in the suicide figures (Moser et al., 1984; 1990). Indeed, the unemployed tend to have much poorer health than those in work (Townsend et al., 1992). This has marked effects on the wellbeing of individuals who are systematically disadvantaged in the light of such circumstances. This may be particularly so among young people. In the words of Platt (1984): 'young school leavers, not being able to find a job, relatively soon develop symptoms of emotional disorders and psychiatric disorders which quickly disappear once a job is found'.

So, we have seen that the characteristics of the general population of those must susceptible to suicide is directly paralleled among offenders. Thus, as practitioners in the criminal and civil justice field, we are highly likely to encounter circumstances where individuals have contemplated or indeed have committed suicide.

Researchers have claimed that suicide rates in prisons are about four times the rates in the community (e.g. Morgan and Owen, 1990; Liebling, 1992; Dexter, 1993). Given the growth in the rate of suicides among those overrepresented in the prison environment, e.g. young unemployed, it is unlikely that the prison environment alone accounts for such differences between community- and prison-suicide prevalence rates. However, despite the overrepresentation of 'high-risk groups' within prisons, prison experience may serve to further increase the risk of suicide. For example, recent research has identified bullying in prisons among young offenders as a major contributing factor to the psychological distress that is so often an antecedent to suicide (Inch et al., 1995). In a prison environment the methods of 'escape' from psychological distress are reduced. The options for young people in prisons if they are being bullied are reduced when compared to outside. Also, if such distress becomes unbearable, prisoners may experience ambivalence about whether or not they wish to share their feelings. This ambivalence may be partly based on the fact that many prisoners when reporting suicidal feelings will be subjected to what Dexter and Towl (1995) refer to as institutionally 'legitimised humiliation rituals'. Their concern is based largely upon a primary focus on physical preventative strategies such as the use of 'strip cells' (often at the expense of a more caring response). This is a concern shared by HM Inspector of Prisons, who clearly stresses the importance of a culture of care being pivotal in suicide management and prevention (Tumin, 1990). A caring response to those who report having suicidal feelings may have the additional benefit of helping others come forward in saying how they feel, reducing the risk of potentially suicidal individuals taking their own lives. There are also a broad range of staff attitudes and responses in prisons ranging from concerned and helpful to those who appear to regard prisoners with contempt (Dexter, 1993). If prisoners perceive the likely staff response to be the latter rather than the former, they are even less likely to report suicidal thoughts and feelings.

A number of themes emerge as precursors to suicide. Loss events (e.g. health, relationships), provocation and frustration, social isolation and alienation may all contribute to suicide. Anniversaries of distressing events may also serve as a factor increasing the risk of suicide. Also, in institutional settings, e.g. hospitals and prisons, a completed suicide may serve to trigger or rekindle suicidal ideas and behaviour in others (Morgan and Owen, 1990). Interestingly, the risk of suicide is highest in the period immediately after admission (into hospitals) or custody (in prisons). This may, in part be directly associated not only with the reasons for the person's admission/custody but with the uncertainty and stresses of a change of life circumstances where there is a high degree of control being exerted over the individual. The rate of suicide is greater in prisons among those held on remand. Broadly, suicide risk in prison increases with the length of sentence.

The sometimes negative views of prisoners held by staff is reflected in their use of language when recording information about suicidal feelings, thoughts and behaviours. For example, terms such as 'attention seeking' and 'manipulative' are used which in effect assign negative motivation to the person's behaviour. Medical staff in particular tend to use such terms as 'threatening suicide'. This may be a more general reflection of pejorative medical parlance, e.g threatening to arrest or abort. However, whatever it is a reflection of, such linguistic practices are singularly unhelpful and in many cases downright dangerous. Assigning negative motivations to an individual's behaviour is generally a poor starting point in trying to help them. Also, if we make all our observations of an individual in line with such prejudices then we may well miss therapeutic opportunities to help reduce the risk of suicidal behaviours.

Thus, we have seen how young male offenders are generally an increasingly 'high-risk group' largely because of their social backgrounds. We have seen also how the prison environment may contribute to exacerbating existing difficulties. Prisoners' difficulties will, to some extent, be accentuated again upon release because of the label of 'ex-prisoner', thus significantly reducing, for example, the individual's chances of getting employment. We have seen how this may affect the personal psychology of the individual (see above, Platt, 1984), thus giving a clear example of the interaction between the social and psychological world of individuals and how they may interact to impact on behaviours.

The psychological context of suicide

Inevitably there will be overlap between the psychological and social context of suicide. This overlap is illustrated in the lists of factors associated with an increased risk of suicide by overdose for young people. These factors include: being male; having a previous history of overdose/self-injury; psychiatric disorder; coming from a large family; disturbed relationships; alcoholism in the family; not living with parents (in young people); chronic problems and behavioural disturbance; alcohol and drug abuse; social isolation; and poor school record (Hawton 1986). Another identified factor may be suicidal behaviour in parents (Pfeffer, 1986).

Depression is a common antecedent mental and emotional state to suicide. Indeed, if we encounter clients who are depressed it is very important as part of our assessment of their depressive state that we make an assessment of their risk of suicide.

Psychiatric disturbances such as schizo-affective disorders, depression and problems with alcohol have been shown to be common contributing factors in suicide. Indeed, some authors have claimed that major depression and alcoholism account for between 57 and 86 per cent of all suicides (e.g. Getz et al., 1987). Those diagnosed as suffering from depression or schizophrenia or alcohol addiction have respective lifetime risks of suicide of 15 per cent, 10 per cent and 15 per cent. Approximately

1 per cent of people who carry out an act of non-fatal deliberate self-harm (DSH) kill themselves the following year (about 100 times the risk of the general population) and 10 per cent of all DSH cases eventually commit suicide. DSH and suicide are thus closely linked (Morgan and Owen, 1990). As we have seen, regrettably, it may often be the case in forensic practice that DSH behaviours are dismissed as 'attention seeking' in a pejorative sense. Such notions may be dressed up in psychological parlance as 'goal-directed', meaning much the same thing. All DSH behaviour should be taken very seriously indeed and not dismissed.

Some researchers (e.g. Shneidman, 1992) have attempted, with varying levels of success, to identify common psychological factors of those contemplating suicide. Shneidman begins by reflecting upon the purpose of suicide, which he maintains is to seek a solution to a perceived crisis or difficulty. Others have also stressed the importance of establishing an understanding of the psychological difficulties that an individual act of suicide was intended to resolve. The common goal of suicide is the cessation of the psychological pains of consciousness. Such psychological pain is the common stimulus to suicide. Numerous authors have argued that it is the understanding of the individual's particular psychologically painful experiences which is at the very heart of helping the suicidal (e.g. Kelly, 1961; Shneidman, 1992). The common stressor in suicide is that of frustrated psychological needs. Thus we may, for example, apply Maslow's model of psychological needs to the suicidal. Briefly stated, Maslow propounded a hierarchical theory of human motivation including attendance to physiological needs, safety needs, belongingness and love needs, esteem needs and the need for self-actualisation (Maslow, 1970). The failure to satisfy such needs, especially those lower down the proposed hierarchy, may well contribute to a resulting psychological state of distress and despair.

This brings us on to the common affective experiences in suicide of helplessness and hopelessness. Numerous researchers and clinicians have pointed to hopelessness as being a key factor in contributing to suicide (e.g. Beck et al., 1979). Often the suicidal individual will have lost all sense of having control or influence over his or her environment (Abramson et al., 1978). The loss of a sense of personal self-efficacy has been linked to poor mental health (e.g. Levenson, 1976; Bandura, 1977; Towl, 1990). Such a collection of experiences are common in clinical depression (Gilbert, 1984).

The common cognitive state associated with suicide, according to Shneidman's typology, is that of ambivalence. This refers to the ambivalent thoughts that an individual contemplating suicide may experience. On the one hand the person may wish to die yet also wish to be saved or rescued.

Perhaps most interestingly, in terms of its therapeutic implications and potential, Shneidman refers to what he terms the common perceptual state in the suicidal, of constriction. This involves experiencing difficulties in maintaining a sense of perspective about the full range of possible options. He refers to understanding such perceptual states as impacting on both affect and intellect. This aspect of the suicidal individual's psychological state is liable to seriously impair their abilities to tap both internal and external (social) resources for more effectively dealing with their problems and distress.

The common action in suicide is escape. Such a person is able to escape or egress by taking his or her own life rather than using other means of escape such as running away or leaving one's husband. As an interpersonal act, suicidal behaviours are frequently characterised by a communication of intent. In 80 per cent of cases from psychological autopsy studies there is clear evidence that there were significant verbal and behavioural clues to the person's suicidal intentions (Shneidman, 1992). Finally, in Shneidman's model we have the notion of consistency in suicide as a style of coping pattern. Here, the practitioner may look to previous experiences that the individual has had where they have felt helpless or hopeless and attempted to resolve their difficulties by escape. However, the evidence for behavioural consistency across diverse environments is, at best, inconclusive (Towl and Crighton, 1995).

RISK ASSESSMENT OF THE SUICIDAL INDIVIDUAL

In making assessments of the likely level of risk of an individual taking his or her life, it is important to preserve a sense of perspective in applying a general knowledge of suicide to the individual case. Thus, what is needed is a synthesis of the nomothetic and idiographic approaches to help inform decision making. In short, what is required is the application of the information and understanding we have about suicide in general to the circumstances (social) and perspective (psychological) of the individual client.

It is important to bear in mind that although many individuals who are suicidal do fall into particular 'high-risk' groups, this is not the case for *all* suicidal individuals. Thus the non-existence of 'high-risk' social or psychological factors by no means excludes the possibility of suicide. The question for the practitioner to answer is not 'Is this person at risk of taking his own life?' But rather 'At what level of risk is this person?' and related to this, 'Is it an acceptable level of risk?'

As with any risk assessment it is often helpful to make explicit the time boundaries of such assessments. This is important because our judgements are generally likely to be more accurate and useful within specified time limits.

The assessment interview

Fundamental to the assessment process is the elicitation of the client's account of events. Specifically, it is important to understand the immediate nature of his or her difficulties, and to get an account of relevant background features. It is worth carefully noting the client's use of language in his or her account of events. We will consider this in more detail later.

The client's account of events and current psychological state serves to inform how the practitioner may proceed in structuring the assessment interview. It is helpful once the client's account has been elicited to check that your understanding of his or her view of the situation and psychological state is accurate. Direct closed questions are also important (e.g. 'Do you feel helpless?'). Further questioning will include a specific enquiry as to whether or not the client has felt or does feel like taking his own life. A matter-of-fact approach is usually most fruitful and supportive. It is important to get a detailed picture of the client's thoughts associated with suicide. Suicidal ideation is linked to suicidal behaviour. However, what is perhaps most important about 'suicidal ideation' is the way in which it is manifest. Dexter and Towl (1995) suggest the following ideational typology for use by practitioners working with potentially suicidal clients.

1 Thoughts indirectly related to suicide, but no evidence of them having considered suicide as a possible or desired option.
2 Thoughts suggesting they would like to commit suicide, but have no intention of carrying it out.
3 Thoughts suggesting they would like to commit suicide, but no evidence of them having made plans to carry it out.
4 Thoughts indicating they would like to commit suicide and they have planned how to do it.

In their research, all the prisoners who fell into categories 3 and 4 of their typology had scores above the cut-off point for Beck *et al.*'s (1975) hopelessness scale (HS). We will give a more detailed description of psychometric tests including the HS in the next section. However, the significance of Dexter and Towl's (1995) typology for the practitioner is perhaps that in the absence of psychometric tests, valid information about suicidal intent can be usefully gleaned using the typology to inform practice.

So, questioning about the degree of reflection, planning and intended method of suicide may elicit useful information in informing the risk assessment process. As a general rule the greater the degree of planning and the more detailed the specification of the method, the greater the risk of suicide.

Also it is helpful to try to get an idea of the duration of such thoughts and their timing. Sometimes individuals will be more likely to contemplate suicide at certain times of day or in particular places. The client should be asked about what reasons they have for taking their life and what reasons (if any) they have for not taking their own life. This information is useful because it gives the practitioner an idea of what inhibition mechanisms the client has in reducing the risk of suicide (Clark and Fawcett, 1992). It is also sometimes worth exploring with the client whether or not their thinking about death includes the death of others. About 5 per cent of homicide cases go on to kill themselves. This is consistent with the observation that there is an overrepresentation, in completed suicides, of those charged with homicide offences on remand in prisons in England and Wales. Most recently it has been noted that those on remand charged with the commission of sexual offences may be at heightened risk of suicide (Suicide Awareness Support Unit, Prison Service, 1995, personal communication).

Table 5.1 contains a list of points to cover in interviewing potentially suicidal individuals. The checklist is by no means exhaustive but rather it is a guide for structuring the interview to ensure that important questions are asked. It is for the practitioner to follow up such areas to ensure that a detailed understanding of the answers elicited has been gained. It cannot be overemphasised that it is important to seek corroborative accounts of events that clients give (e.g. in official documentation or with colleagues or the client's family and friends).

Psychometric testing

It is often helpful to ask the client to complete some short psychometric tests. Although there are a range of tests which may be of use in individual cases, we would advise that as a rule just one or two specialist tests are used rather than broader 'personality type' tests. Five of the most

Table 5.1 Checklist for risk assessment interviews with suicidal clients

1 Ensure that there is a comfortable, private environment in so far as it is possible.
2 Elicit a detailed account of the client's difficulties.
3 Ensure that you have checked with the client that your understanding of their perception of their difficulties is accurate.
4 Ensure that you have a clear idea of their reasoning for taking their own life.
5 Ensure that you have a clear idea of their reasons for not taking their own life.
6 Ask the client if they feel helpless.
7 Ask the client if they have feelings of hopelessness.
8 Ask the client if they have contemplated suicide.
9 Identify which, if any, particular 'high-risk' groups the client falls into, e.g. a young offender being bullied with a history of suicide attempts on remand for a homicide offence.
10 Ensure that you ascertain a clear understanding of suicidal ideation.
11 Ask about whether or not the client has attempted suicide or has intentionally injured themselves before.
12 Assess what levels of social support they have access to.
13 Ask them to describe their activities over a typical day.
14 Ask them which problems are most immediate and pressing.
15 Assess their mood, e.g. depression.
16 Ask about immediate and future plans.
17 Assess impulsivity.
18 Identify those features of themselves or their environment (e.g. social support) which may reduce their risk of suicide.
19 Identify those features of themselves and their environment (e.g. unemployment) which may increase the risk of suicide.
20 Given your overall assessment of the individual and their circumstances identify possible future 'triggers' to suicide which may occur and thereby acutely significantly increase the risk of suicide.

common scales used are: the hopelessness scale; the suicide intent scale; the scale for suicide ideation; the suicidal ideation questionnaire; and the suicide probability scale (Eyman and Eyman, 1992). It is important to stress that psychometric tests can in no way replace the interview. However, some of them may provide very useful supplementary information. Indeed, by observing the way in which the client goes about completing a psychometric test, the practitioner may obtain useful information about the cognitive and affective state of the client.

Beck's depression inventory (BDI) is one of the most commonly used psychometric tests with suicidal clients. It consists of twenty-one multiple choice items which are scored as 0 or 1. This is one of the most researched specialist psychometric tests in the area of depression. It is useful both as a general measure of depressive affect and a measure of possible suicidal intent. Scores of 1 on individual items 2 and 9 on the scale are particularly linked to a higher risk of suicide. Item 2 taps hopelessness and item 9 suicidal ideation. Of course, there is no reason why the practitioner cannot simply ask these two questions as part of the interview process. Indeed, these two items are almost as good as a predictor of suicide as Beck *et al.*'s (1974) hopelessness scale. The scale does, however, suffer from face validity problems for some groups, especially offenders. For example, items 5 and 6 refer, respectively, to feeling 'guilty' and 'punished'. These are often items which may suffer from face validity problems in particular settings. Hence, it is worth the practitioner being mindful of this.

The hopelessness scale (HS) is a twenty-item scale with true/false responses. It provides a better indicator of risk of suicide than the BDI. However, it is worth noting that the scale has only been standardised on adults and not children and adolescents. Hence, this test should only be used with adults.

The scale for suicidal ideation (SSI) is a nineteen-item test designed to attempt to quantify the intensity of immediate conscious suicidal thoughts. It covers five areas: attitude to living and dying; suicide ideation or wish; nature of contemplated attempt; actualisation of contemplated attempt; and background factors (Beck *et al.*, 1979; Eyman and Eyman, 1992).

One major flaw of each of these psychometric tests is that they are easy to fake should the client wish to hide suicidal intentions. Low scores should be regarded with caution and seen in the fuller context of other assessments. However, clearly, some psychometric tests can be a useful way of quantifying progress.

We have surveyed the general area of suicide drawing from nomothetic and idiographic studies. We have followed this survey with an account of how to make an assessment of the risk of an individual client or prisoner taking his or her own life. The next stage of the risk assessment process involves the making of a judgement about the acceptability of the level of risk identified. In general, in making such judgements it may be prudent to err on the side of caution given that suicide is clearly a grave and irreversible act. However, ultimately we cannot be prescriptive on this point except to reassure the practitioner that the making of a full assessment on the lines that we have outlined will help inform such judgements to ensure a fair and just response for the client.

Finally, we would like to stress the importance of careful and close systematic monitoring of individuals identified as being at high risk of suicide. The effective monitoring of behaviour is an essential component of effective risk management across a range of fields (Towl, 1995). Their whereabouts and activities, particularly in more extreme cases, may require close supervision. For the practitioner, on subsequent interviews with the client, it may very well be helpful to rerun through the original checklist from your initial assessment (see Table 5.1) and also to consider re-administering the BDI and HS to provide a quantifiable measure of the individual's comparative psychological state.

SUMMARY

Suicide involves the act of taking one's own life. Comparative research suggests that suicide rates range from 3 to 45 persons per 100,000 of population. In more recent years younger people (aged 15 to 24) have increasingly been overrepresented in the suicide figures. The unemployed are significantly overrepresented in the suicide figures, those who have been unemployed for 12 months are nineteen times more likely to attempt suicide. Such 'high-risk' groups are overrepresented in prison populations. However, despite the overrepresentation of these groups other aspects of such institutionalised life may contribute to the higher rates of suicide in prisons than in the community. For example, bullying may well play a significant role in suicide in prisons for young offenders. Broadly, a number of themes are evident as precursors to suicide: loss events; provocation and frustration; social isolation; and alienation. Anniversaries of distressing events may also serve as a factor in increasing the risk of suicide. Also, especially in institutional settings, e.g. hospitals and prisons, a completed suicide may serve to trigger or rekindle suicidal ideas and behaviour in others. Depression and alcoholism may sometimes be important precursors to suicide. There is also a link between acts of deliberate self-harm (DSH) and suicide. Approximately 1 per cent of people who DSH kill themselves within a year (about 100 times the risk of the general population) and 10 per cent of all DSH cases eventually commit suicide. Suicide ideation can be an important predictor of suicidal behaviours. As a general rule, the greater the degree of planning and the more detailed the specification of the method, the greater the risk of suicide. A number of specialist psychometric tests may be used to help inform our risk assessment decisions with the suicidal, for example, Beck's depression inventory (BDI) and the hopelessness scale (HS). Such tests may be particularly useful as (before and after) measures of therapeutic progress.

Chapter 6

Risk assessment of violence

In this chapter we begin by outlining what areas of behaviour we are mostly concerned with in relation to violent offending, when considering our work as practitioners within the criminal and civil justice systems. We focus on violent crimes, outlining who commits such crimes and under what circumstances such crimes take place. We draw from an understanding of violence to help elucidate those factors which may serve to increase the risk of violent offending. We then consider how such factors may be best applied to individual cases in informing our estimates of the likelihood of such reoffending. Related to this, we examine some considerations associated with the notion of the acceptability of levels of risk in relation to violent offending in informing our decision making.

Violence may take many forms. Probably one of the single most damaging forms of violence is what has been termed 'corporate violence'. Monahan (1981) defines corporate violence as 'illegal behaviour producing an unreasonable risk of physical harm to consumers, employees, or other persons as a result of deliberate decision-making'. He goes on to distinguish between 'street' and; 'suite' violence. He views suite violence as involving corporate violence, for example, poor health and safety at work conditions. He argues that street violence involves people with quite different social and psychological characteristics to those involved in suite crime. Young, black working-class men are overrepresented in the official figures for 'assaults' in the USA. We would add another category to Monahan's categorisation of violence, namely violence within the home. Thus, the reader will be aware that the study and understanding of violence is a politically charged area.

Practitioners in the criminal justice system characteristically encounter those guilty of 'street' and 'domestic' violence. It is because of this that in this chapter we will focus primarily on an exploration and examination of four major crimes of violence: homicide; assault; robbery; and rape. We will examine homicide, assault and robbery in more detail because rape is dealt with in a separate chapter (see Chapter 10).

HOMICIDES AND ASSAULTS

It may be helpful to view most homicides as being at the extreme end of a continuum of assaults. The relationship between homicide and assaults is similar, in this sense, to the relationship between suicide and depression. Just as if we are presented with a client who is depressed and we consider the possibility of him or her being suicidal, we may need to consider the possibility of homicide in clients who have a history of assaults. It is partly for this reason that we deal with homicides and assaults under the same sections below.

Violence, as recorded in criminal statistics, is usually an offence which occurs in the context of someone who offends in non-violent ways too. In a survey of male prisoners in the Southeast of England, Brody and Tarling (1980) found that although only 14 per cent were serving a sentence for violence, 52 per cent had previously been convicted for violent crime at some point in their criminal careers. By comparison, interestingly, in a survey of domestic criminal violence, 16 per cent of women surveyed reported some kind of physical violence towards them over a 1-year period from their partners, and 28 per cent had experienced physical violence from their partners at some point (Gelles, 1982). Intrafamilial homicide accounts for between 20 and 40 per cent of all homicides.

Homicide, rape and assault have in common that both assailants and victims tend to be known to each other (Lester, 1979). The brutal truth is that we tend to be killed, raped or assaulted by people we know. Recent studies on domestic violence serve to highlight this relationship (Dobash and Dobash, 1980, 1992; Dobash et al., 1995). The difference between a case of assault and homicide can often simply depend upon the availability of a weapon. We know that a relatively small number of offenders in general are responsible for a disproportionately large amount of crime (e.g. Farrington, 1993); this also appears to be the case for many violent offenders. Indeed, Lester (1979) maintains that:

'violent crime occurs most frequently in large cities, and is primarily committed by males, especially those between the ages of fifteen and twenty four. Offenders are mainly from the lower social classes'.

However, a good proportion of first offenders are never reconvicted. In one study 14 per cent of those with a first conviction for violence were reconvicted, 40 per cent of those with two convictions, 44 per cent of those with three convictions, and 55 per cent of those with four or more convictions (Walker *et al.*, 1967). However, convictions for violent offending is probably an inaccurate (i.e. massively underrepresentative) estimate of actual offending. But this is likely to be less so in the case of homicide. Indeed, in an early study in the US, 47 per cent of convicted murderers were found to have no preconvictions (Gillin, 1946).

Studies on those who have committed homicide are likely to be more representative in terms of their 'subject sample' than those which seek to investigate assaultative behaviour in general. For example, convicted rapists are unlikely to be representative of rapists in general. Middle-class rapists will rarely face imprisonment. The small subgroup of rapists who serve a prison sentence tend to be predominantly working class.

One area of 'hidden' violence has historically been domestic violence. Walton (1988) defines domestic violence as 'physical and verbal abuse inflicted on women by the men they live with'. Some commentators see domestic violence as a clear example of how patriarchal social norms and policies have served to legitimise domestic violence (Dobash and Dobash, 1980; Wilson, 1983; Walton, 1988). In Scotland, 25 per cent of all violent crimes recorded by the police involve wife assault. Yet in self-report studies only 2 per cent of women who have suffered spousal assault say that they have reported it to the police (Dobash and Dobash, 1980). In Britain, spousal homicide accounted for 40 per cent of all women victims of homicide from 1982 to 1984 (Edwards, 1986). In his review of the literature on the prediction of violent behaviour Monahan states that:

> The research studies on the statistical prediction of violent behaviour have yielded a wide variety of results, ranging from substantially less accurate to substantially more accurate than the studies of clinical prediction, depending upon what criterion of violence was used.
>
> (Monahan, 1981)

In general, statistical predictors of violence are most helpful where base rates are higher. Statistical predictors of low base-rate violence are of little use. A significantly greater quality of information may be gleaned from the individual case. Later, we will go on to examine just how we may make maximal use of both statistical data and our clinical assessments. For the present it is sufficient to note Monahan's exhortation about the importance of the criterion for violence which is used in our assessments.

Homicide tends to be committed by males aged between 15 and 40 (Wolfgang and Ferracuti, 1967) especially by those who are teenagers or in their twenties (Wolfgang, 1967). In a classic study of homicide in Philadelphia, Wolfgang (1958) found that in his 5-year study of homicides, all were committed by blue-collar, lower socio-economic groups. This holds true internationally (Wolfgang and Ferracuti, 1967). Also, homicide and other assaultative crime figures in the US have consistently shown that blacks have rates between four and ten times that of whites. Whereas black couples in the US report spousal abuse at about double the rate for whites (Straus *et al.*, 1980), black children are significantly underrepresented in all child abuse categories. Cross-cultural reviews on homicide have found that there is a greater degree of stability among homicide figures, per head of population for women, whereas figures for men vary greatly. When homicide is committed by middle- and upper-class groups there is a higher likelihood of major psychopathology and/or demonstrable premeditation.

There exists no general relationship between mental disorder and violent crime (Steadman, 1987). Men tend to kill in the street and are killed on the street. Women tend to kill in kitchens and are killed in bedrooms. In short, more homicide occurs inside homes than outside them (Steadman, 1987).

Criminal homicide is usually triggered by escalating altercations, domestic quarrels, jealousy, revenge, arguments over money or robbery. In terms of gender differences in homicide, perhaps one of the most interesting statistics is that wives killed by their husbands account for 41 per cent of women killed, whereas husbands slain by their wives account for only 11 per cent of men killed.

Homicide is a low base-rate behaviour. As early as the 1960s, some commentators were keen to point out that about three times as many people are killed by drunk drivers than are murdered (Morris and Blom-Cooper, 1967). However, in the US homicide is the leading cause of death among younger, lower-social-class males. The highest rates of homicide are reported in Latin America, the Caribbean, North Africa and the Middle-East (Wolfgang, 1986).

But who commits assaults and homicide? Statistical correlates of future violent offending include: previous history of violence, age (15–24), sex (male), 'race' (black), socioeconomic class (low), user of opiates and alcohol and marital status (single) (Monahan, 1981).

Violent crime, as opposed to non-violent crime, is a reasonable indicator of an increased risk of future violent offending. White middle-aged people are more likely to commit corporate crime. The statistical relevance of 'race' once an individual has been recognised as delinquent is non-existent in terms of predicting future violent crime (Wenk *et al.*, 1972). Megargee (1966) has hypothesised that murderous violence may involve two distinct personality types: the undercontrolled personality and the overcontrolled personality. The undercontrolled individual lacks the internal inhibitors which characterise the behaviour of non-violent individuals. The increased impulsivity found among young offenders compared to adult offenders are perhaps overrepresented in the undercontrolled personality group. This group's lack of inhibitive responses, it is hypothesised, make them more likely to respond violently in a range of situations. By contrast, the overcontrolled personality is such that the individual is fastidious in his or her dealings with the social world. The personal psychology of such an individual may be such that emotions, for example, anger, are rarely expressed either physically or verbally. However, such individuals may suddenly, entirely out of character, respond violently to an apparently innocuous 'trigger' to violence. Indeed, one sometimes hears of homicide cases where the perpetrator is described as committing a 'frenzied' attack. Often such media descriptions are juxtaposed with accounts by neighbours of seemingly mild-mannered individuals whom they simply cannot equate with someone who could commit such 'frenzied' attacks. This characterises the Megargee overcontrolled personality type.

Broadly, it is a small group of repeat offenders who commit most violent crime (Toch, 1992). Toch (1969; 1979; 1992) postulated a typology of violent offenders. In his unique study he used ex-violent offenders as interviewers for his investigation into the perspective of the violent offender on violence. Toch commences his account of his proposed typology with his research rationale being that: 'In order to understand a violent person's motives for violence, we must thus step into his or her shoes and we must reconstruct his or her unique perspective.'

According to Toch, two key psychological strategies lie 'behind' why violent individuals behave in a violent way. First, what Toch terms 'self-preserving strategies' and second, 'self-image compensatory strategies'. Self-preserving strategies include reputation defending and norm-enforcing. Reputation defending involves the subcultural acclaim associated with the individual's violent behaviour. Norm-enforcing involves defending a subcultural set of social rules which guide behaviour.

Characterising violence as a self-image compensatory behaviour is the other key element to Toch's typology. The idea is that individuals with a low self-esteem invest time and energy into defending and promoting their feelings of self-esteem. Violence then, is construed as the behavioural manifestation of such feelings. Related to this is the notion that many violent offenders lack social skills, in particular assertion skills, and thus resolve feelings of 'pressure' or conflict by using physical aggression. Such behaviour may involve the bullying and exploitation of weaker others. Toch largely accounts for such behaviour in terms of a need or drive to have control over one's behaviour. Characteristically, individuals with low self-esteem may feel that they have little control over their environment. However, through bullying the individual is able to reassuringly (from his or her perspective) demonstrate control over another.

Toch also outlines two types of orientation that are especially likely to produce violence. One of these is that of the person who sees other people as tools designed to serve their needs, the second is that of the individual who feels vulnerable to diminishment (Toch, 1992). Toch views the former case as accounted for developmentally in terms of the inadequate development of social responsibility during the socialisation process. However, he views the latter case as evidence to suggest that the individual's upbringing has been characterised by insufficient emotional support resulting in difficulty in developing a positive self-perception.

There are some indicators that some features of the home environment can be important in distinguishing between violent and non-violent delinquents. Some of the statistical discriminators include: harsh parental attitudes and discipline; low IQ; and separation from parents (e.g. Farrington, 1978).

It is important to remember that although Toch endorses the notion of 'violence-prone' personalities within his typology, he is aware that: 'Many persons are currently classified as violent offenders who are not really violence-prone.'

ROBBERY

Having looked at some of the social and psychological characteristics of individuals who commit homicides and assaults, we will now turn our attention to examining the characteristics of those involved in robbery.

A number of attempts have been made to provide typologies of robberies (e.g. McClintock and Gibson, 1961; Conklin, 1972; Gabor, 1986). One of the problems in this area appears to be the confusion between 'incident types' and 'offender types'. The early typologies appear to be structured using 'incident' types, e.g. the McClintock typology. More recent conceptualisations have been structured using 'offender' types (e.g. Gabor *et al.*, 1987).

Conklin (1972) devised a typology of robbery offenders based on interviews with sixty-seven prisoners in a Massachusetts prison. About 60 per cent of his sample were black. He distinguished between four 'types' of offender: (1) the professional robber; (2) the opportunist robber; (3) the addict robber; and (4) the alcoholic robber. Professional robbers tend to work in gangs and carefully plan their crimes. They rarely have full-time jobs and in Conklin's sample tended to be white and in their mid-twenties. The largest group in Conklin's sample were the opportunist robbers. This group tended to be young, black and teenagers. The third group, the addict robbers, reported using robbery as a last resort to raise finance to fund their opiate-taking habits. However, this group were particularly characterised by their routine involvement in burglaries, which they viewed as a generally safer way to fund their opiate-taking habit. The final group, the alcoholic robbers, tended to be drunk during the commission of the offence, with little pre-planning.

Robbers who do not carry weapons appear more likely to use physical violence rather than simply to (sometimes implicitly) threaten it. Generally, the reported purpose of robbery is to raise significant sums of money quickly. In this respect robbery is a more efficient crime than, say, burglary. Generally, money gained from robbery can be used immediately, whereas burglaries tend to be characterised by the taking of property, e.g. in house burglaries, taking electrical goods. Such goods have to be sold before the offender effectively can 'make good' his profit from the offence. Thus, one can see how at crisis points a drug addict may be much more likely to turn to robbery to fund his habit speedily.

Most robbers are poor, uneducated and may suffer or have suffered from drug and alcohol addiction problems. They tend to be motivated primarily by monetary gain. Related to this there can be feelings of increased power and control over one's environment as secondary 'motives', although this may be at a conscious or pre-conscious level. Numerous sets of circumstances may serve as precipitants of robbery, for example, unemployment and drug and alcohol abuse. Unexpected additional social or personal stresses may contribute to an increased risk of an individual committing a robbery (Gabor *et al.*, 1987). There are some indications that juvenile robbers tend to spend their 'profits' from robberies on fulfilling their immediate gratifications for drugs, alcohol and parties, whereas, adult robbers tend to be more likely to use the proceeds of their crimes for paying debts and having savings (Gabor *et al.*, 1987). Conklin (1972) concluded from his review of the literature and research into robbery that: 'measures aimed at the reduction of poverty, racial discrimination and relative deprivation will benefit society in many ways, including a reduction in robbery rates'.

ASSESSING THE RISK OF VIOLENCE

We have briefly surveyed homicide, assaults and robbery in terms of some of the things we know about such offences and offenders. We now turn our attention to the situations which may well be important in informing our predictions of the likelihood of an individual committing a further violent offence.

Monahan (1981) cites six types of situational factor which may impact upon the likelihood of reoffending: family environment; peer environment; job environment; availability of victims; availability of weapons; and the availability of alcohol. The practitioner may helpfully assess these areas for an individual in terms of the quality of the former three and the extent of the latter three. Three key questions require addressing in relation to the situations in which the offenders offend (Bem and Funder, 1978), namely:

1   What characteristics describe the situation in which the person reacts violently?
2   What characteristics describe the situations which the person will confront in the future?
3   How similar are the situations the person will confront in the future to those that have elicited violence in the past?

It is worth remembering of course, that 'persons' and 'situations' are not independent of each other. Generally, individuals do not simply stumble upon 'situations', but rather particular situations are features of particular lifestyles. Thus, for example, an offender may complain of being provoked into fighting in pubs. Upon further enquiry into the situation in which such provocations take place, it may be that the pub in question on a Saturday night is known to be a place where fighting is a feature of the evening. In this example the prospective offender would effectively reduce the chances of becoming violent if he or she arranged to visit other pubs (or perhaps the same pub on a different evening or lunch time) where (and when) they would be less likely to encounter such provocations. Also, people will often influence as well as select situations, and the interactionist position within psychological theories of personality clearly emphasises the importance of this interrelationship between the person and situational factors (Mischel, 1968).

THE RISK ASSESSMENT INTERVIEW

In any interview with clients it is essential that there is a clear purpose to the interview. Our assumptions here are that the practitioner is trying to establish:

1 Approximately what level of risk of specific violent offending the individual may present.
2 What features of the individual and their lifestyle is likely to serve to *increase* the chances of them committing specific violent offences.
3 What features of the individual and their lifestyle are likely to serve to *decrease* the chances of him or her committing specific violent offences.

We have seen how statistical studies on the prediction of violent reoffending have shown that a number of social groups and psychological propensities are overrepresented in violent reoffending figures (Monahan, 1981; Toch, 1992). Some researchers have been reluctant to include some demographic predictors of violence such as low socio-economic class on the grounds that such groups are already victimised by society (Ryan, 1971). Whereas we have some sympathy with this viewpoint, not to include such variables in an estimate of the risk of a specific violent reoffending seems to us to be doing a disservice, in particular to potential victims, given that we know that homicide and assault victims are liable to be similar in social characteristics to the perpetrators. Professional practice in the forensic context often involves a weighing up of the rights and (sometimes competing) interests of various interested parties in making our assessments of the individual client. Such ethical dilemmas are not exclusive to the forensic setting. However, they are brought into sharper focus (Towl, 1994c). So, in short, to omit a key variable linked to an increased risk of reoffending would, for us, be ethically untenable.

A number of 'blindspots' for practitioners have been identified when making assessments of 'risk'. First, a lack of specificity in defining the criterion (variable) we are trying to predict. Second, ignoring (statistical data) base rates. Third, relying on illusory correlations and finally, failing to incorporate situational and environmental information in our assessments (Monahan, 1981).

A theme throughout this book has been an emphasis on the importance of being clear about precisely what we are trying to predict. We would add to Monahan's list that such predictions should be time bound. Low base rates, as in, for example, homicide, result in high false positives. This is important because in practice it may mean that we are liable to 'overpredict' the risk of homicidal reoffending. Clearly, an understanding of not only the base rates for the specific target behaviour is important, but also an awareness of the impact of high and low base rates on our predictions. As a general rule it is helpful to make explicit evidence in support of any correlations (e.g. violence and drug dealing), that one uses in informing risk assessments.

A failure to take fully into account situational aspects of a person's lifestyle which may impact on risk is a common error. There is a wide body of psychological literature demonstrating that we have systematic attributional biases in making judgements about the behaviour of others. Overall, we often tend to attribute people's behaviour to dispositional rather than situational factors. Such attributional errors can lead us to miss important situational aspects of a person's lifestyle. An interesting example of the possible significance of situational aspects of reoffending is provided by a study by Bailey (1995) into life-sentenced prisoners, who, after release into the community were subsequently recalled. Lifers who were discharged into the area where they originally committed their index offence appeared to be more likely to be recalled than those who were not. These particular, albeit very tentative, findings may indicate the importance of the general level at which the context of someone's environment may directly impact upon their behaviour.

In summary, relevant factors consistent with impacting upon the risk of violence will include ascertaining the following information: violent history; age; sex; race; social class; opiate and/or alcohol abuse; intelligence; educational attainment; family environment; peer environment; job environment; and availability of victims, weapons and alcohol. Each of these factors require detailed consideration. However, for individual cases often we will simply not have sufficient accurate actuarial data. We are reminded of Meehl's (1973) exhortation that in such cases we should 'use our heads'. In practical terms this means being aware of the limits of the knowledge that we have access to and a clear understanding of its value in relation to the case before us.

Perhaps the single most important factor in predicting future violence will often be the person's history of violence. It is very important to get a detailed understanding of the recency, severity and frequency of specified violent acts. It is wise to seek corroborative accounts of events from relevant documentation, other family members or significant others and professionals. Open-ended questions such as 'What is the most violent thing that you have ever done?' can be helpful. When piecing together the individual's violent history it is sometimes useful to attempt to make a judgement about whether or not the degree and frequency of violent acts is increasing. Monahan and Steadman (1994) suggest that there are three particularly promising 'dispositional markers' of a propensity towards violence – anger, impulsivity and psychopathy. We would argue that, whilst such factors may well require full consideration in individual cases, there is a need to go beyond such 'dispositional' factors.

As we have seen from Toch's (1992) typology of violent men, it is important to explore and examine fully the client's perspective on his or her violence. This cannot be overemphasised. Not only are there many ways of being violent, there are many different reasons for individuals becoming violent. A full individual assessment of the individual's perspective on his or her violence is imperative in helping not only to inform the risk assessment process but also in terms of future treatment implications for reducing the risk of the individual violently reoffending. For example, an individual who is poorly socially skilled but has 'good basic fighting skills' may be more likely to engage in aggressive or violent behaviour because of this combination of skills and skills deficits. One treatment implication to reduce the risk of this individual violently reoffending may be to commence a programme of assertion skills training.

Earlier we mentioned Megargee's (1966) conceptualisation of the psychology of two distinct types of violent offender. It may be helpful to think of these as 'ideal types', in the Weberian sense, when conducting our assessments. For example, an individual who is undercontrolled will benefit from an assessment which clearly specifies examples or evidence for the individual being 'undercontrolled'. Some offenders may be very quick to respond aggressively to the slightest verbal provocation. What would be required here would be a further exploration into precisely what verbal provocations are most offensive for the individual client and, crucially, why (from the client's perspective). Similarly, in the case of overcontrolled individuals, it may be of importance to attempt to understand how clients experience and express their emotions. A potential treatment implication may be to help individuals identify and express their emotions in socially acceptable ways.

Another crucial dimension to understanding violence is the notion of instrumental and angry (or hostile) aggression (Buss, 1961; Toch, 1969; Megargee, 1976). Instrumental aggression is behaviour in which an individual uses violence to get some desired outcome, for example, with robbery, a pecuniary outcome. Angry aggression is where individuals experience anger and become aggressive or violent as a direct expression of their feelings. Where clients appear to be violent as a function of instrumental aggression it may be most helpful to try to aim at working on their core beliefs associated with violent behaviour. However, if clients appear to be primarily experiencing 'angry aggression', then anger management work may be helpful in reducing the risk of violent behaviour occurring (for a detailed examination of anger management treatment work see Chapter 9).

In sum, when attempting to do an assessment of an individual's level of risk of violent reoffending, there is a need to look in detail at the individual's personality and world view, the situations in which he or she is more (or less) likely to offend in and crucially, how the individual's disposition and the relevant situations may interact.

WHAT LEVEL OF RISK OF VIOLENCE IS ACCEPTABLE?

Finally, we will briefly turn to the thorny area of the acceptability (or otherwise) of estimated levels of risk of violence. What we hope to offer the practitioner is a number of considerations which may assist the reader in deciding whether or not a particular risk assessment based on recommendations they make is acceptable. The practitioner needs to address three key issues.

1 *Who is the client?* Earlier we mentioned how the sometimes competing interests and needs of various interested parties need to be taken into account in our risk-assessment decision making. It is worth considering who the various interested parties may be. For example, potential victims have a right to a reasonable level of consideration in terms of their protection from violence, perhaps from our 'client'. It may be that there are particular groups of people who are more at risk of violence from our client than others, e.g. women. It is sometimes a useful mental exercise to take the perspective of each interested party to try to get the best possible overview and understanding that you can of the interests of all concerned in trying to make your recommendations both fair and just.

2 *What are the consequences of an inaccurate decision?* As we have seen there are broadly two types of error which may be made in our risk-assessment decision making – false positives and false negatives. False positives are where we predict that the person is likely to be violent and they are not, within the time frame we have specified. This type of error may raise issues of individual liberty. False negatives are cases where we have predicted that an individual has a low risk of

becoming violent in a specified time period and yet they have in fact become violent. Both types of error are inevitable in the risk assessment process. If we could predict these events with 100 per cent precision then, by definition, there would be no 'risk'. What we seek to do is to minimise the numbers of errors we make and also to attempt to minimise the effect of making such errors. If the practitioner has carefully considered the guidance in this chapter, hopefully it will help to reduce the risk of errors being made.

3 *What are the options?* Risk assessment involves the management of uncertainty. At times we may all find this difficult. However, in risk assessment there is no such thing as a neutral recommendation. Inaction may result in a client being unnecessarily incarcerated or released from prison despite serious concerns. To continue to keep someone in prison, e.g a life sentence prisoner, we may be decreasing the risk of violence to the general public because the individual does not have an opportunity to offend. However, we may also be adding to the person's sense of institutionalisation to a point where he or she increasingly becomes even more difficult to resettle in the community safely.

It is generally important to make recommendations for what should be done for, or with, the individual client when you have completed the risk assessment. Try to examine as many options as possible and use the one that most logically follows from your conclusions.

SUMMARY

Although a great deal of harm and damage is undoubtably done through corporate violence, individuals involved in such activities comparatively rarely find themselves as our clients in the criminal justice system (CJS). Four of the most significant types of violent crime which our clients in the CJS are often guilty of are: homicide; assault; robbery; and rape.

A range of factors have been identified which may be associated with an increased risk of violent reoffending, for example: violent history; age; sex; race; social class; educational attainment; family environment; peer environment; job environment; and availability of victims, weapons and alcohol. It is essential, that when making assessments of the risk of violent reoffending, the practitioner takes a detailed account of the offenders' perspective on their offending (e.g. motivations). Some individuals may be more prone to acting violently than others. Three key questions require addressing in relation to the situations in which the offender may reoffend. What characteristics describe the situation in which the person reacts violently? What characteristics describe the situations the person will confront in the future? How similar are the situations the person will confront in the future to those that have elicited violence in the past?

Part III

Assessment and treatment

Chapter 7

Cognitive–behavioural approaches to offending

INTRODUCTION

In this chapter we will look at the general nature of cognitive–behavioural approaches to problem behaviours. We begin with a short introduction to the history of these approaches and some of the founding principles of both behavioural and cognitive psychology, and the relevance of these to modifying behaviour. This is followed by a general review of cognitive–behavioural assessment and how this can be structured. Finally, we look at some of the general considerations involved in modifying behaviour in this way.

COGNITIVE–BEHAVIOURAL ASSESSMENT

Current cognitive–behavioural approaches to psychological problems have developed out of research mainly conducted since the turn of the century. It was the Russian physiologist Pavlov who elucidated one of the most basic forms of learning, what is now termed classical conditioning. Pavlov showed that dogs could be conditioned to salivate to the sound of a bell if the sounding of the bell had previously occurred when food was given. In this example the food was what Pavlov called an unconditioned stimulus and salivation was an unconditioned response. The sounding of the bell was the conditioned stimulus and salivating in response to a bell was the conditioned response.

Animals put through the procedure showed evidence of a clear learning curve where they began to respond to the bell more strongly with repeated opportunities to learn. They also showed clear evidence of 'generalisation', in that they would show weaker conditioned responses to similar noises (i.e. bells of different tones or pitches). It was also clear that responding to the bell stopped if it was repeatedly sounded without food being given. After a number of such trials the response to the bell alone gradually ceased, a process which has been called extinction (Pavlov, 1927).

A different type of learning was studied in the US by Thorndike, Tolman and Guthrie. They showed in a series of experiments that behaviour which was followed by satisfying consequences was repeated. Behaviour which was followed by noxious or unpleasant consequences was discouraged. They termed this the 'law of effect' (Thorndike, 1932). This work has since been considerably refined and developed, although the basic principle remains intact and is now termed 'operant conditioning'.

These two principles of behavioural learning and their refinements are the basis of subsequent developments in behavioural therapy.

In 1913 another US psychologist John B. Watson argued that psychology should break away from its early emphasis on introspective and philosophical methods, and instead become the scientific study of behaviour. It is for this reason that Watson is often credited as the founder of 'behaviourism' as a separate 'school' of psychology. Watson was also the first to research the conditioning of dysfunctional behaviours. In what would now certainly be seen as an ethically questionable study Watson and Rayner (1920) conditioned a fear response to a white rat in an 11-month-old child. This work was followed up by Jones (1924) who went on to apply Watson's recommendations for reversing this conditioned fear. She discovered that whilst the fear reaction could be reversed, this could only be done effectively by associating the feared object with a pleasant experience (e.g. eating), or by letting the child see other children interact with the feared object without themselves showing fear. Although sadly neglected for many years this research and the methods discovered by Jones are very similar to later behavioural treatment techniques.

Another major development in behavioural therapy was the work of Mowrer and Mowrer in the 1930s into enuresis (bed wetting) (1938). In contrast to analytic methods prevalent at that time they saw enuresis simply as a failure of learning, in this case a failure to respond to bladder distention by waking. This led them to develop an electrical 'bell and pad' system, which woke the child up every time he or she began to wet the bed. This approach proved highly effective.

The name most often associated with the behaviourist school of psychological thought though is that of Burhaus F. Skinner. Skinner renamed the law of effect the principle of reinforcement. He also laid the foundations for much of the research into operant conditioning. Like Watson, he completely rejected the idea of internal mediators (i.e. thoughts and feelings) as legitimate or feasible areas of study. Such 'radical behaviourism' remained the dominant school of thought in psychology until the 1950s; and as such tended to obscure other theoretical approaches.

Even among other behavioural theorists the rejection of thoughts and feelings was never fully accepted. Dollard and Miller (1950), for example, suggested that internal drive states (for example, fear) were needed to explain some learning. They went on to conceptualise and test much of psychoanalytic theory in behavioural terms. Indeed, their work can be seen to have laid the foundations for a broadening of behavioural psychology to encompass findings from cognitive and social psychology.

Another key name in the development of behavioural treatment techniques is Joseph Wolpe. In the 1950s Wolpe, building on earlier research into induced neuroses undertaken by Masserman (1943), studied the conditioning of fear in animals. Later he extended this to fear in people. Wolpe is best remembered for his book *Psychotherapy by Reciprocal Inhibition* (1958). In this book he spelled out a technique which has since been called systematic desensitisation. In essence this involves gradual and graded exposure to a feared object, an approach still used today. Wolpe did this by reciprocal inhibition, essentially the pairing of whatever produced the fear with a pleasant stimulus incompatible with feeling fear. However, the pairing of pleasant and unpleasant stimuli does not as Wolpe thought, appear to be a necessary part of such treatment. Exposure to real-life situations is the most effective way to bring about a reduction in levels of conditioned anxiety.

This work was well received at a time when psychologists were becoming increasingly sceptical about the efficacy of psychoanalytic techniques (e.g. Eysenck, 1952). From this point on groups of applied psychologists, predominantly working in health care settings, went on to develop a range of applications of conditioning theory (see Shapiro, 1961). This led to the development of behavioural techniques to address obsessional behaviours (such as ritual hand washing) and phobias. In the longer term it also gave rise to attempts to apply behavioural techniques to more global problems such as anxiety and depression.

At this time early efforts were also made to use aversion therapy to treat behavioural problems. Aversion therapy involved pairing an unpleasant or noxious stimulus (e.g. an electric shock) with a favoured object or activity. In particular, attempts were made to work on substance abuse problems (especially alcohol abuse) and deviant sexual behaviours. This included disgraceful attempts to 'decondition' homosexual behaviour by using painful aversive stimuli. After much initial enthusiasm the use of aversion therapy quickly declined, both because of concerns about the ethics of using such methods and also because the technique proved ineffective at producing sustained long-term changes in behaviour (Rachman and Teasdale, 1969).

The early 1960s saw a continued growth of the range and use of behavioural techniques in a wide range of problem behaviours. One important technique to mention was the development of token economy approaches. This built on ideas developed by Skinner and Lindsley in the 1950s on the potential applications of operant conditioning (called applied behaviour analysis by them). Ayllon and Azrin (1968) developed a token economy system for a hospital ward for mentally ill patients. Patients earned tokens by behaving in particular ways and exchanged these later for desired goods. The approach became widespread, particularly in North America, and had some success in modifying behaviour. However, more recent research has questioned both the efficacy of the approach and the reasons for any behavioural changes which might be seen. Hall and Baker (1986) suggested that it was increased social reinforcement given by staff rather than the earning of tokens which primarily led to positive changes in behaviour.

Another major advance in behavioural psychology was made by Bandura (1977) who demonstrated the importance of observing and copying others (modelling). Children who observed particular behaviours would copy them without the use of any external rewards or punishments. Bandura and others have argued that such findings cannot be accounted for simply in terms of rewards and punishments for behaviour, and that mediation in the form of thought and language are important in accounting for such copying.

APPLYING LEARNING RESEARCH TO PROBLEM BEHAVIOURS

Applied research into learning followed quite quickly from the pure research, and behavioural methods were at one time widely applied in a range of areas. In applying behavioural research to 'abnormal behaviour' the assumption was often that such behaviours would have been learnt in the same way as more 'normal' or adaptive behaviours. One of the most positive effects of the development of behavioural approaches was to increase greatly the precision with which such abnormal or maladaptive behaviours were described. This included descriptions in terms of magnitude, frequency, rate and intervals between behaviours. Unobservable states such as anxiety needed to be specified in terms of outcomes amenable to observation (e.g. increased pulse rate). Whilst behavioural approaches can now appear to be overly mechanistic they did lay important foundations for understanding what had previously been seen as irrational behaviours. Such an approach also has the great advantage that it set a clear framework within which to evaluate the effectiveness of its own techniques.

This sort of detailed behavioural analysis has led to a great many effective intervention methods being developed. However, it is important to note that because a problem can be treated successfully in a given way using a behavioural framework or approach, it does not mean that the causal explanations offered by behavioural psychologists are true.

COGNITIVE MODELS

Despite the dominance of behavioural models in psychology other approaches did continue to develop and these remained concerned with what is now called cognitive psychology. This term would include language, memory, perception, judgement and reasoning. Perhaps the most neglected cognitive psychologist has been Bartlett (1932) who continued to be interested in cognitive aspects of psychology during the peak of behaviourism. Slightly later Kelly (1955) devised personal construct theory, which stressed the importance of an individual's way of interpreting and understanding the world in terms of 'constructs'. In essence these are discriminations about the world, which give rise to individual patterning of cognitions (Needs, 1995).

Cognitive psychology has traditionally taken a fundamentally different approach from behaviourist psychology. Here, reinforcement of behaviour is seen as secondary or at least cognitively mediated, with cognitive processes being seen as central to behaviour. The whole area of cognitive psychology was reawakened in the 1960s in the face of increasing evidence of the limits of purely behavioural formulations. Attempts to use computer models to simulate cognitive processes also gave a great impetus to the growth of cognitive approaches (see Neisser, 1967).

COGNITIVE–BEHAVIOURAL APPROACHES

One of the main criticisms of cognitive psychology was voiced by one of its leading proponents. Neisser (1976) argued that much of academic cognitive psychology had become overly concerned with pure research and had failed to apply much of what was discovered to problems with real significance outside the laboratory. Although at this time applications of cognitive psychology were developing with the use of problem solving, covert imagery and self-statements to problem behaviours.

The current cognitive–behavioural synthesis represents the application of research findings from cognitive psychology. Overall, the approach represents a break from behavioural formulations in that it assumes an important, and usually dominant, role for cognitive processes such as thoughts and feelings. However, practitioners working in this way use both cognitive and behavioural methods, acknowledging that behaviour can be one of the most powerful tools for changing the way a client thinks about something (see Bandura, 1977).

COGNITIVE–BEHAVIOURAL ASSESSMENT

This is based on principles derived from experimental psychology. The main idea here is that a person's behaviour will be influenced by the outcomes of the behaviour and that such behaviour is mediated by cognitive processes (i.e. thoughts, feelings and memories).

Accordingly the purpose of a cognitive–behavioural assessment is to develop an initial formulation of a client's problem or problems. These can then be tested and refined over time and in the light of experience. This will involve educating the client into the idea that the process is an active one on their part, which will involve them in analysing and resolving their own problems with the help of the practitioner. This may often be complicated by the nature of forensic populations, who frequently present with multiple problems, i.e. alcohol abuse, aggression, family problems. In addition, forensic clients may be undergoing treatment work on a mandatory rather than a voluntary basis. This is likely to reduce the number of positive treatment outcomes since initial motivation is likely to be lower in many cases.

As with any other group of clients, we would argue that initially an essentially sympathetic and concerned approach is usually most productive. It is especially important that forensic clients are assessed to ensure that emergency intervention is not required (e.g. clients in custody who may become actively suicidal).

Assessment

There are a variety of techniques which can be of value in undertaking a cognitive–behavioural assessment. The main methods are listed in Table 7.1.

Table 7.1 Methods of cognitive–behavioural assessment

1 Structured interview.
2 Self-report questionnaires.
3 Self-monitoring of behaviour (diaries).
4 Behavioural observation ratings.
5 Physical measures.

Some of these methods might only be used occasionally, either because they are not relevant to a particular case or because of practical problems in taking the required measurements. Interviews and self-monitoring are fundamental aspects of this approach and will generally be used. Other self-report measures are also frequently used and we will look at each of these in turn.

Interviewing

The basics of a cognitive–behavioural interview will differ little from other approaches to interviews, and many similar considerations will apply. Specifically, clients will generally value adequate privacy. They will need to have, or develop over time, a level of confidence in the practitioner. Practitioners may also find it helpful to have adequate background knowledge about an individual client and to build up an appropriate rapport with them.

It can be useful to begin an assessment by getting clients briefly to outline their perspective on their problems. This can serve the useful function of giving practitioners an estimate of motivation and insight. It is likely that any work which does not begin from this starting point will be less effective than it could be.

Whilst the client's perspective is an essential starting point, it is seldom if ever detailed enough. Practitioners will generally want to build on this basis. In general we would advocate an essentially supportive and constructively critical approach to a client's problems during assessment, rather than being either confrontational or uncritical. This is because the aim of assessment is to analyse the client's problems in detail and in realistic terms. Openly confronting offenders in the initial stages of assessment tends to make a detailed analysis more difficult. Confrontation may be necessary in some cases but is generally more effective only once an adequate understanding of an offender's difficulties has been established. Prior to this the results of direct confrontation can be more entrenched denial. In contrast, a totally uncritical approach may result in perceived collusion with distorted ideas and beliefs. These ideas and beliefs may then become harder to challenge effectively later. Clearly the balance between information gathering and challenging is a matter for individual judgement. We would in most cases argue that the assessment phase should emphasise the former even at the expense of the latter.

Whilst the cognitive–behavioural approach focuses primarily on current events, it is often useful to conduct a review of the development of a problem over time, since this can give useful clues about the events which precede, and the outcomes of, particular behaviours.

Below we outline a framework for cognitive behavioural interviews. We would stress that this should not be seen as set in stone. The different aspects of the interview schedule can be seen as largely interchangeable and the precise progression will be largely dependent on the practitioner and client's sense of priorities. However a good assessment would include information on most or all of these areas (see Table 7.2).

Table 7.2 Interview schedule

---

1   Brief outline of current problem(s) from the client.
2   Outline of problem development.
3   *Problem(s)*. Description of each problem area in terms of thoughts, feelings and behaviours, i.e. What? When? Where? Who? How?
4   *Maintaining influences*. Situations, emotions, thoughts and the behaviours of the client and others which may be involved in maintaining the problem(s).
5   *Social factors*. Family and other relationships along with other factors such as accommodation, occupational and social contacts.

Having gathered this information it should then be possible to formulate some ideas about why a client is having particular problems based on a cognitive–behavioural framework.

Below we apply the interview schedule in Table 7.2 to a case example of an offender being supervised, and receiving treatment, in the community.

Name: John
1   History of excessive use of alcohol over the last 5 years. Currently on remand for burglary which he started to finance his drinking.

2 *Age*   *Behaviour*
   12   First drink.
   14   Regular drinking with friends.

16   Hospitalised with alcohol poisoning.
16–19   Stopped drinking completely.
19   Girlfriend left. Started drinking again. Charged with being drunk and disorderly.
20   Charged again with being drunk and disorderly.
        Charged with resisting arrest and drunk and disorderly.
21   Charged with burglaries (five). Remanded for reports.

3 Started drinking again at age 19 when he broke up with his girlfriend. Initially went out with friends to pubs and clubs, or drank cans of lager in the shopping centre with friends. Later drinking in the morning at home to reduce hangovers. Prior to arrest drinking all day until money ran out. States that drink helped him to socialise. That he generally felt lonely and bored before drinking. He also said that he felt stupid not drinking when his friends felt, that 'real men' could hold their drink.

4 *Situations*   Social situations. With friends who all drank and encouraged him to do so.

   Behaviours   Everyone else drinking. Later began to get the shakes and drank to stop these.

   Emotions   Felt very happy when drunk. Self-confidence much better and able to speak to people well.

   Thoughts   This is better than being alone at home. I enjoy being happy. My mates will think I'm a tosser if I don't drink. You only live once.

   Physical effect Stopped the shakes.
                    Hangover but a drink reduced this.
                    Sometimes sick.

5 *Social factors.*
   Previously in local authority care and foster homes. Currently living in a council flat on a large estate. Lives alone. Unemployed, previously on schemes but the last one ended a year ago. No hobbies or interests outside the pub. Feels he is not confident enough to mix without a few drinks.

From this point the practitioner might have some initial ideas about why John drinks heavily. For example, it appears that he lacks social contacts, therefore boredom may be a factor. He also seems to lack confidence and uses alcohol as a way to overcome this. These sorts of ideas can often best be tested by getting clients to self-monitor their thoughts, feelings and behaviour in a diary.

Self monitoring

This can take a variety of forms but diaries are most frequently used. One of the benefits of this is that it gives useful information for the practitioner to evaluate, and where necessary change or refine, their initial ideas about a problem. Returning to John, an extract from a self-report diary which he was asked to keep is shown in Table 7.3.

By getting clients to record their thoughts, feelings and behaviour over time it is possible to get a much better picture of a client's problems, and the processes involved in maintaining these. This in turn makes it easier to see the areas where help is most needed and most likely to be effective in changing the problem behaviours. There are also clear problems with getting clients to record their behaviour and thoughts. One of these is that clients may not be motivated to keep such detailed recordings. This often can be overcome by carefully explaining the reason for using the approach, and stressing that the intervention is a collaborative approach. More practical considerations such as literacy can be important also. Here, one solution is to use tape-recorded diaries, rather than written ones.

In addition to getting the client to self-monitor their thoughts and behaviour it may, in some cases, be possible to get other people to monitor a client's behaviour. This is generally more feasible in residential settings such as hospitals, prisons or bail hostels. For some problems, friends and relatives can be of assistance to the client in helping them monitor their behaviour.

Self-report measures

These are frequently used and generally take the form of questionnaires about an individual's thoughts or behaviour. As such they can supplement information gleaned from the interview and as such may help give a better understanding of a client's problems. The main difference here is that some questionnaires allow the responses of one client to be compared with those of a large number of others, in turn giving some idea of how specific or general their problems may be. They can also be of benefit in allowing a comparison of responses before and after treatment, giving some idea of how effective this has been. There are though also drawbacks in using questionnaires. Most crucially there is a weak relationship between the results of many questionnaires and actual behaviour (Mischel, 1968).

Table 7.3 An example of a self-report diary

Time	Behaviour	Situation	Thoughts	Feelings (How strong 0 to 10).
9–12	Asleep until 11.30. Got up and had a drink of water	At home/in the flat	Tired. Got nothing to do all day What's on TV?	Irritated 2 Bored 3
12–3	Watched TV	Flat	This is rubbish	Bored 4
3–6	Watched TV	Flat		Bored 7
6–9	Went down to the pool hall. Met up with Andy and Daz	Pool hall with mates I'd known from school	Pleased to see my mates. We might have a laugh. This is better than being at home	Cheered up 6
9–12	Went into pub. Had a few pints of cider. Tried to chat up the barmaid	Duke of York in the town centre	Pleased to be out – got something to do. This is a good laugh. Wish I always felt this good/confident	Happy 9 Confident 8
12–3	Took a bottle of cider home with me. Drank it when I got back to the flat. Crashed out at about 2.30	Flat – on my own		Relaxed 8

COGNITIVE BEHAVIOUR MODIFICATION – SETTING PRIORITIES

Cognitive behaviour modification (CBM) subsumes a variety of cognitive and behavioural techniques which can be used by a practitioner. We will cover some of those which can be effective for particular problems in forensic settings in later chapters. In Table 7.4 we list some of the best-known techniques.

Table 7.4 Cognitive–behavioural techniques

Cognitive therapy	Beck, 1967; 1991
Cognitive restructuring	Ellis, 1962
Self instructional training	Meichenbaum, 1972
Anxiety management training	Suinn and Richardson, 1971
Problem solving training	D'Zurilla and Goldfried, 1971

Such intervention techniques differ in several respects. First, they will involve different strategies for intervention, ranging from direct confrontation of ideas to more gentle Socratic methods of challenging ideas. Here, the approach would be to explore carefully the ideas and evidence which support particular ideas. This evidence can then be analysed and challenged as a way to reduce belief in the original idea.

Second, the approach offers a number of points at which the practitioner can intervene in what Meichenbaum (1976) termed the 'cognition – affect – behaviour – consequences sequence'. Finally, different methods will focus on different aspects of cognition: some will challenge basic beliefs and belief systems, others will involve coping self-statements and so on.

However, CBM approaches have some key features in common which distinguish them from other types of intervention. First, all such approaches must actively involve the client in addressing and solving their own problem(s). Second, all are very structured approaches, and will always be time bounded. By this we mean that both client and practitioner will work within a clear framework which involves the client in actively testing out the effectiveness of other ways of thinking and behaving. This will be quite different from many clients' expectations of being 'cured' of their problem(s).

CBM can be seen as having four main objectives:

1 To improve a client's level of understanding and insight into their problem behaviour(s).

2 To enable clients to think about their cognitions (e.g. thoughts, mental images) and to learn to see these as ideas which are themselves worthy of testing – rather than simply accepting them as facts.
3 To encourage clients to undertake behavioural experiments which will often produce evidence which contradicts existing ideas, and to consider their cognitions in the light of these.
4 To equip clients with new cognitive and behavioural skills.

CBM can be seen as a framework and also a range of techniques which help practitioners to achieve these aims.

Cognition is the term used to describe mental events, and in turn these can be broken down into events, processes and structures.

Cognitive events

These are the thoughts and images that we can experience and are sometimes described as 'internal dialogue'. A great deal of human behaviour does not seem to involve internal dialogue at all. For example, few experienced car drivers conduct an internal dialogue about how to drive a car, although they may engage in other sorts of internal dialogue. Such behaviours have become largely automatic or 'scripted'. However, for a significant amount of time we do seem to engage in such 'self-talk' and this in turn seems to influence the way we feel, behave and evaluate the outcomes of our own behaviour.

Meichenbaum (1977) suggests that such conscious self-talk will naturally occur when an individual:

1 Attempts to construct and integrate new action sequences.
2 Has to exercise choices in novel situations.
3 Anticipates or experiences an intense emotion.

Cognitive processes

This term refers to the automatic ways in which we all process incoming information. For example, we are all selective, and indeed have to be so, about what we attend to in our environment and how we appraise it. An example of this might be the heavy drinker who pays attention to the locations of pubs and off licences in their local area.

Problem solving can also usefully be mentioned under this heading. Some forensic clients are generally poor at problem solving. For example, they may be very impulsive and so spend little time processing information but instead, acting immediately (Needs, 1995).

Cognitive structures

These are a theoretical aspect of cognition and have been variously termed schemata (Piaget, 1932), 'blueprints for thought and actions' (Neisser, 1976) and 'meaning systems' (Meichenbaum, 1977). At their simplest these terms are used to convey the idea of selective 'templates' of thinking, which in turn influence how we appraise events. So, for example, an obsessional individual might have an overall 'meaning system' which states that it is crucially important to do things perfectly all the time. Clearly such overall beliefs are likely to influence behaviour greatly.

Changing behaviour

As mentioned earlier, CBM starts from the premise that in order to get long-term and lasting changes in behaviour, we need to produce changes in the cognitions which maintain these behaviours. Whilst it has proven possible simply to behaviourally condition people not to behave in particular ways, such changes have often not been sustained. In other cases, attempts to modify behaviour, without working on cognitions, have simply not worked at all (see Williams, 1994). Therefore in CBM the primary emphasis has been to increase the client's awareness about thoughts, feelings and behaviours and their consequences (including their impacts on others).

In practical terms this involves attempting to interrupt and change existing, and often largely automatic, patterns of thinking. This begins with developing an awareness of thoughts in terms of events and also processes. Some techniques used in CBM will also address cognitive structures. In addition, many clients will need to be taught a variety of behavioural and cognitive skills to help them function more effectively. These skills will in turn need to be tested. Finally, in CBM we would suggest that there is a need to structure client's expectations about lapses. Partly because the cognitive–behavioural approach is essentially one of self-management, such lapses will almost inevitably occur. The approach of 'relapse prevention' is often portrayed, quite wrongly in our view, as an optional extra to a cognitive–behavioural intervention or alternatively as an intervention procedure in its own right. It is more constructively seen as an essential aspect of an effective cognitive–behavioural approach (see Pithers, 1990).

Metacognition

This term was used originally to refer to an individual's awareness of their own cognitive processes. Early research was concerned with memory but this has since been extended to include studies on the self-control of behaviour, communication and peer relationships (see Meichenbaum, 1977). What seems clear from such research is that much of individuals' 'internal dialogues' are, in general, not at a conscious level. It seems that individuals can use a greater awareness of their own internal cognitive processes to improve control over their behaviour. The best-known example of this is self-instructional training (Meichenbaum, 1972; 1975) and the application of this to anger management in both individual casework and also groupwork in prisons (Towl, 1993; 1994a, b).

OVERVIEW

For the purposes of description it is possible to outline CBM in terms of a series of stages. It is rare for any intervention to proceed smoothly from one stage to the next. It is much more common for clients to move between stages as the intervention progresses. In broad terms the process can be divided into three main stages:

1 Developing the client's understanding of the problem by means of a collaborative effort.
2 An exploration of the presenting problem(s).
3 Modification of the reciprocal interactions between thoughts, feelings and behaviours.

To take each in turn, clients will usually have some conceptualisation of what their own problems are. How far these agree with the views of others will vary greatly. It seems rare that clients will see the role of their own thinking processes. It is also rare that people see the extent to which thoughts, feelings, behaviours and outcomes influence each other. For example, individuals who believe that everyone is likely to attack them are likely to become generally tense and angry at the prospect of impending attack. This in turn may lead them to become hostile towards others, who in turn may become aggressive towards them. Many people do not clearly see the role that their own reactions play in maintaining maladaptive behaviours.

The first goal in a cognitive–behavioural intervention is therefore to involve the client in a collaborative effort to investigate the problems they experience. As already discussed this will involve detailed interviewing, and also the use of self-report measures such as diaries of behaviour and thoughts and possibly also questionnaires or other measures. It may also involve the practitioner setting homework in the form of behavioural tests or experiments for the client to try.

As in assessing the client, the process of intervention is not simply an uncritical acceptance of what the client's interpretations of events are but an effort to explore and test these. The aim being here to reformulate some of their maladaptive interpretations into more adaptive ones.

This can often be greatly facilitated by using a group-based approach and this is something we will advocate in many of the succeeding chapters. This is because it is often easier for other group members to see the transactional nature of someone else's thoughts, feelings and behaviours. In forensic settings it is also often the case that other group members can be very effective at challenging maladaptive ways of thinking, and suggesting other credible alternatives. This credibility in turn often rests on the experience of particular subcultures that group members have. As a rule practitioners will have little experience of the subcultures which many offenders may come from.

At this stage intervention is also concerned with the development of insight, in particular into ideas which may be contradictory, not supported by logic or evidence and which may be self-defeating and in some cases self-fulfilling. Aspects of a client's thinking may be linked to particular problem behaviours. For example, the client who believes that they are constantly under threat of unprovoked physical assaults may be more likely to behave in an aggressive way towards others. This is often where self-monitoring is most useful since it allows the practitioner to identify and draw out these aspects of functioning. It also provides concrete examples which can then be explored and challenged with the client.

The next step is a consolidation of ideas about the problem(s). This can involve identifying any recurrent themes which seem to span several areas of an individual's life (for example, the importance of control, equity and social acceptance). Such themes can have a major impact on behaviour.

Behaviour during group or individual sessions can also be an important focus which can be used to promote positive changes. For example, the non-participation of a client during a group session can be constructively used. Whilst caution may be needed it is possible to probe what the individual concerned is feeling and then ask how those thoughts and feelings might make it difficult for them to participate. From there, it is then often possible to begin to test how accurate or relevant these thoughts and feelings might be. So, for example, clients who do not speak in a group intervention might think that others will think they are stupid if they ask questions or make points and that because of this, other group members will dislike them. It may in this case then be possible to make explicit the links between thinking this way and becoming too anxious to think. The accuracy of such thoughts, in terms of anticipating the thoughts and responses of others in the group, could be tested out with the group. In this case the response might be that they may feel some questions to be stupid and some not; they may also feel that they all ask daft questions sometimes, that many of the other group members wanted to ask that question but were thinking the same things.

From this point, it is often possible to link back what has been discussed to the agreed therapeutic rationale. So in this example it would be possible to go back to the main theme, that our thoughts and emotions influence the way we behave. Here the individual was clearly thinking in ways that made it more difficult for him or her to participate in the group. The next link that could be made is to try out other ways of thinking which might make it easier for him or her to participate. For example, other people also feel anxious. 'I'm not stupid for asking questions, it's the only way to find out things.' 'Other people in the group might want to know this.' In a group setting it is often possible to elicit these statements from the group. Individual work may require more help from the therapist but again the aim is to collaborate in producing credible alternatives that the client feels able to at least try.

The main point here is that it is often not the external quality of events which is important and which produces reactions such as anger or anxiety. Rather, it is frequently the individual's interpretation of events which is critical in giving rise to dysfunctional emotions and maladaptive behaviours.

SUMMARY

In this chapter we have outlined some of the main points in the historical development of the cognitive–behavioural approach to intervention work. We have also given an outline of some of the main principles in conducting assessment and treatment work using cognitive-behavioural techniques. The main assumption of the approach, based on a considerable body of experimental research, is that thoughts, feelings and behaviour all interact with each other to produce observable behaviours. The aim of cognitive–behavioural interventions is to allow these features to interact in a way which allows clients to function as effectively as possible. With forensic populations this will generally mean ways which enable them to reduce their risk of reoffending.

In the following chapters we will look at some of the main areas of application of cognitive–behavioural psychology with forensic populations. The main points covered apply to all these areas, which essentially involves a tailoring of these methods to address the needs of particular problems.

Chapter 8

The assessment of anger management difficulties

INTRODUCTION

In this chapter we consider the nature of anger and give guidance on how practitioners may assess clients who may experience anger management difficulties. Concomitantly, we structure our examination to address issues of risk assessment linked to anger management difficulties.

Practitioners in numerous areas of the criminal and civil justice systems will no doubt be aware of an apparent upsurge of interest in anger management interventions. For example, there has been a considerable growth in the area of anger management groupwork in prisons in the 1990s (Towl, 1993, 1995). In a recent national survey, anger management groupwork accounted for 10 per cent of all groupwork undertaken in prisons (Towl, 1995). This is probably an underestimate of the true level of anger management groupwork undertaken. This is because this study only invited reports of exclusively anger management groupwork as a discrete area of intervention. However, it is evident that a number of other areas of groupwork may also include components of anger management work, for example, sex offender treatment work and offending behaviour groups.

It seems likely that anger management work will continue to be a growth area throughout the 1990s within forensic settings. There are some significant signs of expansion in the prison service, for example, the next major national 'treatment programme' in the Prison Service in England and Wales due to come on stream shortly will be designed for violent offenders. This is likely partly to involve the application of anger management interventions (HM Prison Service, 1995a).

However, despite such growth in interest and practice of anger management work it seems that there remains a great deal of conceptual confusion and potentially ill-informed practice in this area. Below we seek to contribute to reducing such confusion and hopefully to provide a helpful and readily applicable guide to the assessment of anger management difficulties. We begin by addressing one or two fundamental questions.

THE EXPERIENCE OF ANGER

What is anger?

Anger is an emotion. Often the term anger is used interchangeably with aggression. We view aggression as a behaviour. We believe that it is very important to distinguish these two terms in this way. We further detail the characteristics of anger below. However, having identified anger as an emotion, it is valuable first to consider anger in the general context of emotions.

One of the earliest theories of emotion in psychology was the James–Lange theory. This theory dates from the end of the nineteenth century. Briefly stated, they maintained that unpleasant stimuli are responded to by an increased state of physiological arousal resulting in the experience of emotion. For them, physiological arousal was a necessary condition of emotional experiences.

One problem with their theory was that physiological arousal *per se* may precede a number of different emotions. This would seem to suggest that emotions are not solely the result of increased physiological arousal. At the beginning of the twentieth century, Cannon argued that emotion producing stimuli result in two independent bodily systems being activated. One system is the autonomic nervous system (ANS) which results in increased physiological arousal. The other is a perceptual process whereby the brain interprets external events resulting in possible emotional states (Cannon, 1915). The commonly referred to 'fight or flight' reaction to emotionally arousing stimuli roughly corresponds to emotional responses of anger or anxiety, respectively.

During the 1960s these two theories were substantially developed and revised. The importance of cognitive mediation in emotional states is now widely acknowledged (e.g. Arnold, 1960; Schacter and Singer, 1962; Lazarus, 1966). In other words the way we interpret events and our experiences is important in determining whether or not we become angry. The role of our cognitive appraisal of events has become a central notion in current theories about emotion.

Some have been critical of the emphasis on cognitive mediation in the experience of emotions. For example, one objection has been that often anger is triggered very quickly, so quickly that it seems unconvincing to believe that a great deal of cognitive mediation has been involved (Zajonc, 1980). Interestingly, this is a view often put forward by clients who experience difficulties in managing their anger. We believe this criticism to be based upon a highly restricted and misleading definition of cognitive mediation. The criticism takes scant account of attitudes and beliefs. We contend that our beliefs and attitudes may often play a significant role in influencing what sorts of things anger us.

There are two distinct yet related types of cognition involved in the mediation of emotional states. A link between emotional responses and environmental stimuli and personal goals and beliefs (Smith and Lazarus, 1993). One potentially difficult area which emerges from such postulations of the role of cognitive appraisal is the issue of whether or not, or to what degree, one is conscious of such appraisal processes. An analogy may be drawn with, for example, everyday experiences of covert racist behaviour. One may intellectually reject racism but practise it albeit without the intention to being racist. Thus, one may experience being afraid or emotionally aroused if approached by a group of black youths in a way that would be less likely to happen were it a group of white youths.

Emotions other than anger such as depression and anxiety have generally attracted a great deal more clinical and research interest (e.g. Beck, 1991). Later we will see that by drawing from work on other emotions we may enhance our undertaking of anger management difficulties too.

We have seen how emotions involve us making evaluations of our social and inner mental worlds. Two critical components of emotional experiences involve an alteration of our readiness for action and an awareness of the appropriate phenomenological tone felt or experienced as part of the emotion. The experience of emotions often involves a conscious preoccupation with relevant events, bodily 'disturbance', i.e. great activity or inactivity and various bodily expressions of emotions, e.g. smiling or feeling happy (Oatley, 1992). Thus, our emotions are part of our understanding or meaning that we attribute to ourselves and our social worlds.

What are the functions and features of anger?

Functions

Perhaps the most influential figure in the development of anger management work is Raymond Novaco. Central to the development of his treatment work in anger management is an understanding of the 'functions' of anger. He views anger as having six functions: (1) energising; (2) disrupting; (3) expressing; (4) defending; (5) instigating; (6) discriminating. The energising function is manifest with the increased amplitude of responses experienced. The disrupting function may be understood in terms of anger having the effect of both inducing impulsivity and interfering with rational thought processes. The expressing function is characterised by angry individuals communicating what they are angry about. The defending function is associated with the protection of one's ego. Novaco's fifth function of anger, 'instigation' may be seen when anger is followed by aggression. Thus anger may instigate aggressive behavioural responses. Finally, anger may serve a discriminating function, for example, in the definition or appraisal of events as provocation (Novaco, 1975).

Features

Novaco has further developed his conceptualisation of anger (e.g. in Novaco and Welsh, 1989) to include a broader consideration of social information processing. Novaco and Welsh argue that provocation episodes may be most helpfully understood in terms of information processing errors and perceptual or behavioural 'scripts' for anger and aggression. What does this mean? It may be helpful here to draw a parallel with people who are experiencing depression. A number of theorists have argued that depressive states are characterised by a number of characteristic 'faulty cognitions', sometimes referred to as 'musturbations'. For example, everyone *must* like or love me. This is clearly an unrealistic expectation. However, such beliefs if checked against experience may well result in further feelings of depression because the terms of the belief may well not be met. So, to return to anger, we may have unreasonable beliefs about the world which may increase the risk of us experiencing anger. Further to this at an attentional level, we may 'seek out' events which anger us. We may also have experience of close links between anger and aggression. Novaco refers to these processes as 'attentional cuing' and 'perceptual matching'. Thus, we attend to certain events and match them with our past experiences. Such a conceptualisation is based upon a general model of 'pattern recognition'. For example, Mr X is in a pub and a gang of youths in one corner of the pub become increasingly rowdy and drunk. This may elicit a general process of 'pattern recognition' for 'trouble', i.e. an increased risk of Mr X becoming angry with and aggressive towards the said youths. However, at this point, we would wish to emphasise that anger is not a necessary or sufficient antecedent to aggression. Oftentimes individuals may be aggressive without being angry, e.g. in a boxing match or when mugging someone. Some researchers have helpfully distinguished between what may be termed 'hostile aggression' and 'instrumental aggression'.

In the literature (e.g. Spielberger *et al.*, 1995) such acts are sometimes referred to as instrumental aggression, that is, aggression linked to an explicit sense of purpose, in our examples to win the boxing match or to get money from the victim of the mugging. Instrumental aggression contrasts with what is sometimes referred to as 'hostile aggression', i.e. aggression directly linked to precipitative angry feelings. This is an important distinction to be aware of particularly when, for example, later considering selecting clients to participate in anger management work. It is, of course, a very common human experience for people to become angry without becoming aggressive.

A fundamental assumption 'behind' information processing accounts of human behaviour is that few, if any, situations in adult life are approached in a truly novel manner (Nisbett and Ross, 1980). Potentially anger-provoking events are no exception to this. Thus, pattern recognition of potentially anger-provoking events involves making a comparison with previous experiences of potentially anger-provoking stimuli.

There are various biases in such mental processes. Five such biases may be particularly pertinent with information-processing models, namely: attentional cuing; perceptual matching; attribution errors; false consensus; and anchoring effects. We will explain these sequentially.

Attentional cuing involves attending to specific events based on past experience. People with difficulties in managing their anger may ruminate mentally about prospective anger-provoking situations (Novaco, 1986). This may serve further to show their selective attention towards potentially anger-provoking stimuli.

Perceptual matching involves a mental process whereby one compares previous experiences or 'patterns' (of interaction) with the current environment or patterns. Generally, the more exposed individuals have been to anger the more likely they are to perceive anger. Of course, this needn't necessarily be problematic. We shall return to this point later when giving a more detailed account of the assessment process (Novaco and Welsh, 1989).

One attribution error, sometimes known as the fundamental attribution error, is that individuals have a marked tendency to overattribute dispositional factors at the expense of situational factors when accounting for the behaviour of others. For example, a bank robber may get angry with a member of the bank staff for not having a set of keys for a safe, during the commission of a robbery.

False consensus is perhaps one of the most common information-processing biases. False consensus refers to the assumption that everyone would endorse views similar to one's own. For example, Mr Y believes that if anyone makes jokes at his mother's expense he may legitimately become angry and assault the individual who is responsible for the joke. Mr Y believes that everyone else would experience a similar level of anger and express it assaultatively. Such beliefs may be reinforced within particular subcultural settings, thus making them more resistant to change.

Anchoring effects refer to the phenomena whereby our initial judgements and assessment of individuals or situations are resistant to change even when subsequent information calls into question our initial impressions. As suggested by earlier theorists (e.g. James, 1890; Cannon, 1915; Arnold, 1960; Schacter and Singer, 1962) anger generally involves (feelings of) heightened physiological arousal. In effect, such increased autonomic nervous system activity may increase the risk of the individual behaving aggressively partly because the body is physiologically prepared 'for action'. The role of anger as a precipitant of aggression has been advocated (e.g. Berkowitz, 1962). Interestingly this link between anger and aggression may also operate in the opposite direction. Some researchers have argued that any factor that increases the likelihood of an aggressive response will also increase the likelihood of anger (Stearns and Stearns, 1986).

THE EXPRESSION OF ANGER

It is very important to distinguish between the experience and expression of anger (Towl and Dexter, 1994; Spielberger et al., 1995). In the preceding section we outlined some features and functions of anger in terms of the experience of anger. We have seen how anger is one of a number of emotions, characterised by high arousal levels and particular cognitive patterns. In this section we look at the related issue of the expression of anger. Often anger may be constructively motivated. In one study 63 per cent of subjects reported that their 'motive' for anger was to assert their authority or to improve their image (Stearns and Stearns, 1986). Using Novaco's earlier mentioned functional typology of anger we can see that the function of anger for these subjects may have been, in part, as an instigator for assertion. 'Angry behaviour' is frequently habitually inhibited. Non-aggressive behaviour is very common when angry. Impulses towards verbal aggression are reported as being about as common as impulses towards physical aggression. Perhaps one of the more common manifestations of the expression of anger is through the denial of particular benefits which may be seen as a relatively highly socialised form of aggression. This can, of course, be a deeply unethical way to express anger.

One of the key difficulties experienced by many offenders is in the appropriate expression of their anger. Experimental studies tend to provide support for the notion that women and men experience much the same levels and types of anger in response to similar stimuli (Averill, 1982). However, some differences in the way that women and men express their anger have been reported, although the evidence in the area of gender differences in the expression of anger is by no means conclusive (Spielberger *et al.*, 1995). The research in this area tends to suffer from a general, lamentable tendency to conflate emotions with behaviour. For example, 'women are not entitled to anger . . . except in some girlish tantrum' (Bardwick, 1979). However, a number of interesting findings have emerged. Women are more likely to cry when angry than men. Women report feeling hurt more often when they are the target of the expression of someone else's anger. Perhaps the most common form of aggressive anger expression is between spouses. In the United States almost a third of married couples report physical violence in their relationship (Straus *et al.*, 1980). Similar figures have been obtained from studies in New Zealand. In another study it was reported that those men who seriously assaulted their wives but were 'under-controlled', seriously assault others too. Whereas those men who seriously assaulted their wives but are 'overcontrolled', tended to be violent more or less exclusively to their wives. The latter group also tended to report more frequent and intense feelings of guilt (Subotnik, 1989). We shall return to the significance of the 'overcontrolled' and 'undercontrolled' distinction in the next chapter because there are a number of direct treatment implications for such assessments.

So, in sum we have seen how anger is a common and normal human emotion. However, anger may be more or less well managed. Poor anger management strategies may result in physical and mental ill-health of the individual and those who may be affected particularly by aggressive angry expressions.

THE ASSESSMENT INTERVIEW

We have seen how some researchers conflate anger and aggression in their studies. This confusion may well be reflected in the referrals for assessments that practitioners may be faced with. Personal safety should be one important consideration when interviewing potentially violent clients. People referred because others believe that they have anger management difficulties are a potentially volatile group. It is extremely important to be aware of the fact that during the assessment process the client will be expected to talk about their experience and expression of their anger. When giving such accounts clients may well become annoyed or angry again simply as a result of the process of recounting memories of anger. It is partly for this reason that it is especially prudent to break down the assessment interview into manageable chunks.

You may wish to ask the client to complete a psychometric test, e.g. the state trait anger expression inventory (STAXI) (Spielberger, 1988). The interview may begin with a general exploration of what makes the client angry. A 'what? where? why? who with? when? and how?' questioning sequence may be helpful in speedily ascertaining an over-view of the anger experiences of the individual.

What?   It is important to invite as many responses as possible. One way of facilitating this process can be to ask, 'What is it that has made you most angry?' and then to ask, 'What are the sorts of day-to-day things that annoy you?' The task then becomes to fill in the details of anger experiences between these two extreme conditions. Another (and possibly complementary) method is to ask the person to talk through what had angered them over the preceding month.

Where?   Building upon the assessment information from the preceding section, invite clients to detail where they become angry, e.g. in the home, in pubs. Ask where the most common place in which they become angry is located. Ask where they have not become angry.

Why?   This is probably the single most important aspect of the assessment process, namely eliciting an understanding of why the client becomes angry, from his or her perspective. Information in response to this area of questioning will have very clear implications for informing the treatment/intervention process. Follow-up questions are important here. For example, some clients report that they get angry because they feel that others are not showing them sufficient 'respect'. Ask such clients to give a number of examples of this happening. Explore further what they view as 'sufficient respect'. Above all, get as detailed an account as is feasible to help inform the assessment process most fully.

Who with?   We have seen how people most commonly report getting angry with those closest to them. It may also be that certain 'types of people', e.g. authority figures, more frequently precipitate feelings of anger in clients. It is important to elicit who such people are. It is helpful to ask for examples of where specified individuals or 'types of people' have contributed to the client's angry feelings.

When?   Again it is useful to get a picture of how predictable, or otherwise, the timings of a client experiencing anger are. This will be important in helping contribute to the structure of possible treatment interventions.

How?   This is the set of questions which will help establish precisely how clients *express* their anger. We have seen that commonly anger remains unexpressed externally. However, internally we have seen how individuals may be thinking about verbally or physically aggressive put-downs of the target of their anger. Some clients will demonstrate a very clear and robust link between their feelings of anger and aggressive behaviour. Ask what are the most aggressive things they have ever done and ask about their most common acts of aggression. Follow up with questions asking for examples and details.

Once you have elicited a full account of the individual's experience and expression of anger in the context of their lifestyle and social circumstances, explore his or her level of motivation for behavioural change. You may also wish to consider whether the client would benefit most from groupwork or individual casework.

ANGER DIARIES AND SELF-MONITORING

You may wish to ask the client to keep a daily anger diary. This is especially helpful for those who will go on to do treatment work. It is important that the diaries are structured to elicit the most relevant information. See Table 8.1 for an example of how a diary entry for a single day may be structured. The diary is on two sheets with three separate sections. Sheet one is a record of the general level of anger experienced by the individual at three set points during the day. Sheet two contains two sections, one on the client's experience and expression of anger in relation to specific events or situations which have occurred during the day and the other on the anger-management strategies and skills used during the day. All clients will have something to record in the first section of the day's diary entry and many will have information to put in either sections two or three or both. The information provided on such sheets may be a significant aid to both the forensic practitioner and client in understanding the particular anger-related difficulties experienced by the client. This forms an essential assessment base from which to inform judgements about the most appropriate type, and application of, anger management methods. Also the act of self-monitoring may well have an impact on decreasing perceptions of anger related events and improving anger management methods through practice and self-reflection.

Table 8.1 Anger diary

Sheet 1

---

1 *General 'anger' ratings*
  First thing in the morning
  Time . . .

not at all angry	moderately angry	extremely angry

  Mid-afternoon
  Time . . .

not at all angry	moderately angry	extremely angry

  Last thing at night
  Time . . . .

not at all angry	moderately angry	extremely angry

Sheet 2

---

2 Examples of *experience* and *expression* of anger
  Experiences of anger today
  What?
  Where?
  When?
  Why?
  Who?

  Expression of anger today
  How?

3 *Anger management strategies used today*
  Before   Practice of methods and planning for possible difficulties
  In   Methods used in the situation
  After   What did I learn from this?

WRITING ASSESSMENT REPORTS

As with any reports it is important to be mindful of the needs of the target audience. Be clear in distinguishing between opinion and fact and be explicit about your evidence for assertions made. For our purposes we will assume that the report is structured to help inform treatment intervention decisions. Hence, include comment on: the motivation of the individual, a detailed account of their experience of anger (see the preceding interview structure) and their expression of anger. Include details of the frequency and intensity of both the experience and expression of anger. Throughout the report be explicit about the client's cognitive patterns which you deem most relevant to his or her difficulties. For example, the earlier mentioned notion of 'false consensus' whereby the client assumes that everyone would, say, express their anger in much the same way they do, may be of great help in informing specific treatment targets. It may be helpful to look back through the earlier section in this chapter on 'What are the functions and features of anger?' for some ideas about what sorts of characteristic cognitive patterns may be germane.

SUMMARY

There has been a significant growth in anger management work in forensic settings in recent years. Effective anger management inter-ventions have been characterised by a cognitive–behavioural approach.

The term 'anger' is often confused or conflated with the term 'aggression'. Anger is an emotion, and as such is perhaps best understood in the context of theories of emotion. A critical distinction which may be made with anger is between the experience and expression of anger.

As an emotion anger may have both positive and negative aspects to it, largely dependent upon how it is managed, or ultimately expressed. Raymond Novaco cited six functions of anger: (1) energising; (2) disrupting; (3) expressing; (4) defending; (5) instigating; and (6) dis-criminating. Further research work has focused upon the nature of the cognitive processing associated with the experience and expression of anger. Women and men tend to *experience* similar levels of anger. However there is some evidence to suggest that they *express* their anger differently. Broadly stated, men may tend to externally express their anger (i.e. at other people or objects) and women may tend to internalise their anger.

The assessment interview involves eliciting a detailed account of the client's experience and expression of anger. Anger diaries may be used as a component of assessment information to help inform further the development and implementation of later treatment work.

Chapter 9

The treatment of anger management difficulties

In this chapter we begin with a brief introduction to anger-management treatment work. Then we move on to the main focus of the chapter, i.e. giving an examination of practice issues including planning, exercise content and processes, evaluation and the management of role plays.

INTRODUCTION

In the 1960s significant progress was made in delineating and developing our understanding of the emotions. The seminal work of Schacter and Singer (1962) on the role of cognition in the experience of emotions has been influential in the development of successful interventions for people experiencing emotional difficulties such as anxiety (Meichenbaum, 1972), anger (Novaco, 1975) and depression (Ellis, 1976).

Three major components form the mainstream of anger management programmes. First, treatment objectives aimed at the increased awareness and regulation of physiological arousal. Second, a set of treatment objectives aimed at promoting a greater awareness and control over cognitive dimensions to the experience of anger. Third, a set of treatment objectives aimed at focusing upon behavioural strategies to improve anger management skills, for example, assertion skills. Perhaps one of the hallmarks of a good programme is the effective integration and application of these three components (Novaco, 1975, 1986; Novaco and Welsh, 1989). Listed in Table 9.1 are intervention techniques which are commonly used on anger management programmes (e.g. Prison Service National Anger Management Programme 1995b) (HM Prison Service). The relative weighting of treatment techniques directed at Arousal, Behaviour and Cognitive factors, respectively will depend to some degree upon the assessment information gleaned.

Table 9.1 Interventions for anger management

Psychological component	Intervention Techniques
Arousal	Relaxation training
Behavioural	Role play, e.g. of assertion skills
Cognitive	Cognitive reappraisal techniques

ANGER MANAGEMENT GROUPWORK – HOW TO DO IT

In this section we will cover organisational, selection, planning, debriefing and evaluation issues. Then we will outline a selection of exercises and details of how they may be facilitated. Finally, we examine a number of common difficulties which may arise in undertaking such work. Our primary focus in this final section is in giving pointers to assist the practitioner in anticipating and ameliorating difficulties to help enhance the treatment programme.

ORGANISATIONAL AND PLANNING ISSUES

It is important to have an awareness of the political context in which practitioners work. Anger management groupwork does not occur in a social vacuum. In criminal justice systems practitioners are likely to be acutely aware of the increasingly politicised nature of their work at a number of levels. In practice, this awareness will be helpful in informing judgements about how the work fits into the agency or organisational setting. We would not wish to be overly prescriptive about this area. However, it is potentially important because if full consideration is not given to such basic organisational issues, the whole programme may be undermined. A number of questions which may be helpful at this initial stage would include the following. Who else other than the identified client will be affected by the client's participation? Who else is working with the client? What, if any, other work is being done, and how does this intervention fit in with it? Who will need to be informed of the work? How does the work fit into the priorities of the organisation or agency? What level of management support will there be? Once it is agreed and understood precisely how the groupwork will 'fit into' the organisational context, a number of very practical organisational arrangements need to be clear. A brief checklist is given below.

Checklist for planning anger management groupwork: practical resources and arrangements

1 Locate an appropriate venue.
2 Be clear about how long sessions will be and when the group will meet.
3 Establish who the group facilitators will be.
4 Decide upon what is going to be included in the programme.
5 Arrange time to review precisely how the programme will be implemented.
6 Establish how and when the selection of candidates will take place.
7 Ensure that a maximum of ten people are in the group.
8 Agree how the group will be evaluated.
9 Brainstorm possible practical problems and generate a range of possible solutions.

Considerations in the selection of an appropriate venue would include ensuring that there is plenty of space, that the participants will be comfortable and that there is easy access to the venue.

The spacing of the sessions is important. Facilitator and client availability are primary considerations here. Also, in terms of the groupwork the spacing of sessions will have an impact. Broadly, the greater the interval between sessions, the greater the opportunity for clients to undertake 'homework assignments', which are important. However, the closer the sessions, the easier it is to maintain and develop a sense of group cohesion. A rate of two to three sessions per week may be about the right balance for session spacing in view of these two biases.

It is probably best to have two facilitators when undertaking anger management groupwork. This is because it is demanding work which requires a high degree of sensitivity and awareness to the needs of participants.

When deciding upon a programme of anger management groupwork, try to look at as many examples as possible. We strongly recommend that programmes should include exercises to help clients deal with their anger-related arousal, behaviour and cognitive appraisals. Above all, ensure that the exercises you select are relevant and focused to the needs of the individuals in the group.

Setting aside time to talk through the logistics of precisely how each exercise will be facilitated is very important indeed. There are usually many different ways in which exercises could be run. Much of the finer detail of such planning is probably best left to the debriefing sessions once the work is underway. This way the facilitators may be more sensitive and receptive to the specific needs of the group.

It is absolutely essential that an effective method of selection is used. We strongly recommend that all prospective candidates are individually interviewed. Prisoners referred for anger management groupwork should:

1 Acknowledge that their anger management methods have room for significant improvement.
2 Express a willingness to talk about their anger management difficulties in front of others with similar difficulties.
3 Express a desire to change and further develop their anger management methods.
4 Express a willingness, and demonstrate their ability, to contribute constructively to a group respecting the rights of others.

It may be helpful to ask the prospective candidate, at interview, to give a detailed example of their difficulties with anger management. Ideally, full assessment information will already have been obtained. In practice this may be rare. In addition to the guidelines given above, just as with any groupwork intervention when selecting candidates, it is worth considering the 'mix' of participants. For example, it would probably be unwise to select only those people with major anger management difficulties with very aggressive interpersonal styles. This could place group members at risk by substantially increasing the likelihood of violent behaviour within the group. On the other hand, one would not wish to have a group of very overcontrolled individuals who said little. Always ask prospective candidates if they anticipate any difficulties in attendance. It may be helpful to give the client a structured anger diary (see our example in Chapter 8) for completion between the time of the selection interview and the first session of the group. As a general approach it is useful to go through your interview structure with the client as part of a matching process. In other words, explain what is available, emphasise that you are assessing its suitability for the client as much as his or her suitability for it. Thus, the interview is concluded by making a decision about the suitability for the groupwork in meeting the client's needs.

Generally, it is understood in the groupwork literature that between six and twelve candidates for groupwork interventions is about right as an environment to ensure the best opportunity of a group functioning effectively (e.g Brown, 1989). In anger management work, we feel that ten should be the limit because of the intensity of the work.

The effective evaluation of groupwork is notoriously difficult (Crighton and Towl, 1995). Anger management groupwork is no exception to this. However, we contend that it is, or perhaps more accurately should be, part of the programme to build in an evaluation.

Evaluation studies (e.g. Towl and Dexter, 1994; Smith *et al.*, 1995) have included the use of psychometric tests, Spielberger's (1988) state trait anger expression inventory (STAXI) and Novaco's (1980) anger scale, respectively. Some evaluative work has been undertaken with more qualitative measures involving, e.g. structured interviews to ascertain whether or not (women) participants have improved their anger management strategies and skills (e.g. Cundy, 1995). Behavioural checklists may also be used to compare participants' expression of their anger before and after the groupwork intervention. In prisons measures of institutional compliance such as the numbers of disciplinary reports awarded before and after such work have also been used.

The brainstorming of possible problems is an important exercise to go through to enable facilitators to circumvent them.

THE FIRST SESSION

As a general rule in groupwork the first session is the most anxiety provoking for all concerned. First impressions count. Both facilitators and clients benefit from the social investment involved in the selection process. Familiar faces take the edge off anxieties. Information gained during the selection interview may form the basis of informal interaction (and dialogue) whilst the group is assembling.

An essential task in the first session is the spelling out of the group rules. The principles include making clear precisely what is expected of the clients. Equally, it is important to spell out what service is on offer. When making explicit what is 'on offer' it is important to include an overview of the groupwork and its purpose. The course is divided into three parts:

1 Exploring anger.
2 An individual examination of anger.
3 Anger management methods

Each part requires a high degree of participation from the group. The aim of the course is to help clients increase their control over their anger. The facilitators need to make a statement of their commitment to the work. They also need to stress the individual responsibility of each group member for what they get out of the group. The inclusion of a cliché such as 'You will get as much out of this group as you put in' is generally well received. It serves to structure expectations in the direction of a high degree of participation by clients.

Group rules must include basic logistics, e.g. the number (and times) of sessions and also the venue. Stress the need for punctuality – this cuts both ways – facilitators will need to arrive on time too and be well prepared, allowing time for last-minute preparations and the setting up of equipment (e.g. flipcharts). There is little enough time. Make a statement about the fact that all clients have been selected because of their suitability and commitment to the work. The whole group benefits from each individual's contribution. It is important to outline the boundaries of confidentiality within (and without) the group. The expectation is (as agreed at the selection interviews) that participants will attend *all* sessions. However, it is recognised that within some environments, this is sometimes not possible for good reasons. If anyone is unable to attend a session it is essential that they discuss this with the facilitators beforehand. It is not acceptable for anyone to miss a session without having informed the facilitators. Generally, where this happens we would advise that the person is removed from the group. Basic democratic principles of interaction will also need to be spelt out, e.g. everyone is entitled to express their opinions and have the opportunity to be listened to. It is useful to emphasise the benefits of working as a group, e.g. the benefits of joint understanding and problem solving.

N.B. Make it clear from the outset that the bulk of anger management methods outlined and suggested during the group are taken from a number of similar previous groups. The facilitators cannot offer 'solutions' but rather 'suggestions' which others with similar difficulties have found useful.

The facilitators sometimes may find it helpful to say something about how, within the groups, not all suggestions of anger management methods will be effective for everyone, but past experience has shown that everyone will find some suggestions of use. Ensure that everyone is given the opportunity to ask questions or clarify any points.

During the facilitation of the first session it is especially important to encourage all to participate. This does not mean that everyone has to say something. Verbal contributions provide a helpful indication of someone's level of involvement in the group but so do non-verbal responses, e.g. smiles and nods of agreement or acknowledgement. The facilitators do need to try to ensure that everyone who appears to want to contribute verbally has the opportunity to do so.

Thank the group for their attention/participation at the end of the session.

EXERCISES FOR ANGER MANAGEMENT GROUPWORK

This selection of groupwork exercises derived directly from clinical work (see Towl, 1995) falls under three headings.

1 Exploring anger.
2 Individual examination of anger.
3 Anger management.

Each exercise in each of the three sections begins with a 'content aim' and 'content objectives' followed by a 'process aim' and 'process objectives'.

The content aim and objectives provide the practitioner with guidelines to work through the structure of a given exercise. The content aim is a general statement of what information needs to be conveyed during the exercise. The content objectives guide the reader in a more detailed consideration of how to meet the content aim.

The process aim and objectives are principles for the practitioner to take account of and work towards during each exercise. The process aim is a general statement of what underlying principle to work at in each exercise. The process objectives specify practical ways of achieving the process aim.

So, in sum, the content aim and objectives give the exercises some basic structure. The process aim and objectives provide principles to link into group discussion. Finally, exercise briefs are outlined.

EXPLORING ANGER

Exercises I, II and III are facilitated using the ubiquitous flipchart, a selection of coloured felt tip pens and copious quantities of adhesive putty. It is helpful to keep all the materials generated in the exercises in full view throughout the sessions. Such materials may be referred back to during sessions, especially to illustrate learning points and remind the group of the ground covered. Facilitators may use these materials as cues to explore points raised in more detail or simply to clarify particular points.

Exercise I

Content aim

To explore 'anger'.

Content objectives

1 To get an indication of what *situations* group members associate with high potential for a loss of control over their anger.
2 To get an indication of what *thoughts* group members associate with a loss of control over their anger.
3 To get an indication of what *feelings* group members associate with a loss of control over their anger.

Process aim

To elicit a sense of group cohesion and individual involvement.

Process objectives

1 To encourage as many responses as possible at each stage of the exercise.
2 To point out commonalities and acknowledge individual differences in contributions elicited.

Exercise brief

The word **ANGER** is written at the head of a sheet of paper on a flipchart.

1 Group members are asked to say what *situations* they associate with anger. Typical responses include pubs, nightclubs and at home.
2 Group members are asked to say what *thoughts* they associate with anger. Typical responses include, 'He's taking a liberty', 'I'll show him', 'The bastard', 'He's ignorant', 'I'll put some manners on him' and 'If I don't hit him he'll think I am a soft touch'.
3 Group members are asked to say what *feelings* they associate with anger. Typical responses include: frustration, hatred, tension and jealousy.

Exercise II

Content aim

To convey that the negative consequences of losing control over anger outweigh the positive.

Content objectives

1 To show that positive consequences tend to be short term.
2 To show that negative consequences tend to be long term.

Process aim

To establish a sense of group consensus.

Process objectives

1 To encourage everyone to acknowledge a negative consequence of a loss of control over anger.
2 To encourage everyone to acknowledge a positive consequence of a loss of control over anger.

Exercise brief

Group members are asked to list the *good* and *bad consequences* of losing control over their anger. Typical responses include: (for *good*) release of tension, feelings of satisfaction, a problem solved, shows strength of feelings; (for *bad*) imprisonment, deprived of family and friends, creates more problems, it's more likely it will happen again, people may get hurt and things might get out of hand.

Exercise III

Content aim

To outline a graphical model of anger experiences.

Content objectives

1 To indicate that our susceptibility to a loss of control over anger fluctuates over time.
2 To indicate that we may be aware that our underlying levels of anger may increase over the course of a sequence of events.
3 To indicate that certain events may act as 'triggers' to our feelings of anger.

Process aim

To get the group to identify with the model.

Process objective

To use participants' contributions from earlier exercises to illustrate the model.

Exercise brief

A model of anger is outlined graphically in Figure 9.1.

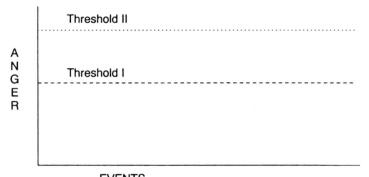

Figure 9.1 A model of anger

The vertical axis represents levels of anger experienced. The horizontal axis represents events which may result in an increase of (sometimes underlying) feelings of anger. The broken lines labelled thresholds I and II represent fluctuating day-to-day tolerance levels to anger-provoking stimuli. When an individual's threshold level at a given time is passed, control over temper is lost.

The facilitator links the model to the general and/or specific comments about anger already elicited from group members. So, in the personal accounts given earlier in the group, any awareness of a build-up of underlying anger or general fluctuating tolerance levels to anger-provoking stimuli need to be explicitly linked to the model. Making a start here may involve saying something like:

> John, you mentioned earlier that a number of things were beginning to wind you up before you lost your temper. Could you remind me of some of those things again, so that we can try and see how it all fits in on the graph.

INDIVIDUAL EXAMINATION OF ANGER

During the 'individual examination of anger' exercises, the dominant activity from the facilitators' viewpoint is in establishing a detailed individual assessment of the anger management problems of each group member.

Exercise IV

Content aim

To elicit detailed individual accounts of anger management difficulties.

Content objectives

1 To break down accounts into a number of discrete (although directly linked) events.
2 To clarify what, if anything, happened between identified events.
3 To encourage the group to ask questions of clarification for each individual account given.

Process aim

To demonstrate that the loss of control over anger tends to be part of a largely predictable set of circumstances.

Process objective

To encourage an awareness of the links between the sequences of behaviours and events which result in a loss of control over anger.

Exercise brief

1 Group members are asked to go into pairs. Each member is asked to give the other an account of a situation involving their loss of control over anger. It is important to give some structure to such accounts in terms of suggested subheadings. For example, the *background* to the *situation, thoughts* and *feelings* at the time of the event and *consequences.*
2 Each person is then requested to give the account of events that they have been told by their partner in the exercise. Key issues are identified

and written up on the blackboard/flipchart. It is advisable to 'check out' the account with the other member of the pair. Also, it is particularly important that you ensure that you have a sufficient understanding of the event outlined. This is important because such information is critical in making a full assessment of each individual's anger management difficulties. An incomplete or inaccurate assessment is likely to result in inappropriate suggestions for specific anger management methods.

3 Once each group member's account is up on the blackboard/flipchart they are analysed by the group. The facilitator initiates the analysis for each account by asking the group 'At what point was there no turning back?' 'Why was this?' Disagreements or differences of opinion about the answers to such questions are examined further in discussion. In terms of structuring the discussion the facilitators cannot go far wrong (!) if they keep the discussion within the labels – the background, situation, thoughts, feelings and consequences. Although at this stage it is probably not necessary to 'fit' reported experiences directly with these labels, it is important to have a general idea of the significance and meaning of events for individual group members. The facilitators must clarify their understanding of the reasons 'behind' individual group members' answers.

Exercise V

Content aim

To outline the BIA (Before, In and After) model of anger.

Content objectives

1 To link the BIA model to the graphical model outlined in an earlier session.
2 To illustrate the BIA model using examples from accounts already elicited from individual group members.

Process aim

To encourage an understanding of a straightforward framework for the subsequent generation of anger management strategies.

Process objectives

1 To emphasise the importance of self-awareness in anticipating potentially difficult situations at the *Before* stage.
2 To emphasise the need to have a set of strategies to use *In* anger-
provoking situations.
3 To emphasise the need for self-reflection, self-criticism and/or self-
praise at the *After* stage.

Exercise brief

Introduce the BIA model of anger. It is essential that when introducing
the BIA model, examples are used to illustrate the three stages. Where
possible and appropriate, use examples previously given by group
members. Explain that:

1 *Before* involves self-awareness, the anticipation of events and practice
or rehearsal of anger management skills (i.e. relaxation, coping self-
statements).
2 *In* involves the awareness that things may be getting out of hand and
using certain strategies and skills to cope with the situation.
3 *After* involves self-reflection, self-criticism and/or self-praise.

Distribute handouts on BIA. Encourage discussion in exploring the BIA
model in terms of the individual accounts given by the group members.
Link BIA to the earlier used graphical illustration of the manifestation
of anger (see Exercise III).

Exercise VI

Content aim

To promote an understanding of the effects of beliefs on behaviour.

Content objectives

1 To encourage group members to list a number of relevant beliefs.
2 To encourage group members to make explicit the links between their
beliefs and behaviour.
3 To suggest possible links between identified beliefs and behaviour.

Process aim

To develop an awareness that beliefs are not 'given' facts and that they may be subject to scrutiny and reflection in the light of their influence on behaviour.

Process objectives

1 To encourage critical self-reflection on the link between beliefs and behaviour.
2 To encourage the exploration of differences in beliefs.
3 To emphasise the consequences of holding particular beliefs.

Exercise brief

Ask group members to share their beliefs which are associated with their loss of control over their anger. Always give examples, e.g. 'If someone insults me, I have to stop them getting "one over" on me/taking the piss.' Use examples given by group members to identify core beliefs which are linked to the loss of control over anger. You may wish to talk through or role play a carefully considered example to illustrate the link between beliefs and behaviour. Towl (1994a) cites the following helpful example. A man (Harry) is in a pub with his girlfriend. Men at the next table are swearing. Harry says to the men at the next table, 'Keep down the swearing – there's a lady present.' This comment may be indicative of the following core belief: *Men should not swear in front of women in public.*

In the group discussion the facilitator encourages the exploration of beliefs. It is essential *not* to remain neutral about particular beliefs and sometimes to challenge certain beliefs.

Exercise VII

Content aim

To convey the range of physical symptoms of beginning to lose control over anger.

Content objective

To encourage the group to list physical symptoms of their loss of control over their anger.

Process aim

To increase self-awareness of the physiological manifestation of anger.

Process objectives

1 To encourage the exploration of commonalities in physical symptoms experienced.
2 To encourage the acknowledgement of individual differences in physical symptoms experienced.

Exercise brief

Ask group members, 'What are the physical symptoms of beginning to lose control over your anger?' Typical responses include – shaking, increased heart rate, increased rate of breathing, sweating palms and a general feeling of 'boiling over'. List all the responses on a flipchart/blackboard. Emphasise commonalities in experiences and acknowledge individual differences.

ANGER MANAGEMENT

Exercise VIII

Content aim

To outline the applicability and relevance of the BIA model in formulating and using anger management strategies.

Content objectives

1 To encourage group members to apply the BIA model to examples of their successful anger management.
2 To encourage clients to generate anger management strategies for each other using the BIA model.
3 To illustrate the BIA model in suggesting possible anger management strategies.

Process aim

To provide group members with a straightforward conceptual framework to help them develop and explore effective anger management strategies.

Process objective

See 'content objectives' above.

Exercise brief

Reintroduce the BIA model stressing the importance of self-awareness and the anticipation of difficult situations. In this exercise the idea is to focus on the situational aspects of individual accounts given. Here you may usefully refer back to and encourage the development of responses given in Exercise I, for example, pubs, nightclubs, home. It is sometimes helpful to get the group to rank a number of situations – which facilitators and other group members may generate – in terms of their potential for the loss of control over anger. The avoidance of 'high-risk' situations is explored and sometimes advocated. At all times encourage, acknowledge and develop alternative ways of dealing with identified situations. This exercise involves a great deal of thought about practical suggestions for 'alternative management of situations'. Facilitators are well advised to think through a number of positive practical suggestions before commencing this exercise.

Exercise IX

Content aim

To demonstrate the applicability of 'self-talk' strategies in anger management.

Content objectives

1 To encourage group members to list a number of self-talk statements which may be of use *In* anger provoking situations.
2 To suggest self-talk statements which may be of use to particular individuals in the group.

Process aim

To get group members to acknowledge and apply self-talk strategies in negotiating their way out of potentially anger-provoking encounters.

Process objectives

1 To ask group members to recount what they have said to themselves in cases of their successful anger management.
2 To ask group members to recount what they have said to themselves in cases of their unsuccessful anger management.
3 To emphasise the major role of 'self-talk' in critical situations.

Exercise brief

Introduce the notion of 'cognitive self-talk techniques'. Rework examples given in the earlier exercises (e.g. Exercise IV) with the group. Scrutinise the examples in terms of possible 'self-talk' strategies to help each other deal more successfully with such situations. Typical examples of self-talk techniques used are:

1 I am in control of my anger.
2 I am not going to let this person/event make *me* lose *my* temper.
3 Maybe it's best to pause and think for a moment before I speak.
4 Perhaps it's better to say nothing here.
5 I must be careful about the tone of my voice.
6 I must be careful what words I use to say what I mean.
7 Maybe it's best to get out of this situation. I will go.

After getting group members to list a number of 'positive self-talk statements', for the examples earlier generated by the group, the facilitator completes the exercise by asking group members to rank the self-talk statements in their order of usefulness to each individual in the group. Advocate the notion that group members have a number of different self-talk statements. Sometimes it may be helpful for group members to use 'prompt cards' of statements which could be used before going into anger provoking situations.

Exercise X

Content aim

To outline the use of Relaxation Training (RT) as an effective anger management tool.

Content objectives

1 To ask group members to clench their fists and then completely relax their hands.

2 To distribute RT handouts.
3 To encourage suggestions for the control over physical symptoms, e.g. by going to the gym.

Process aim

To emphasise and develop feelings of control over physiological responses in critical situations.

Process objectives

See 'content objectives' above.

Exercise brief

Relaxation training (RT) is introduced in this exercise. Group members are encouraged to employ relaxation techniques to counter the physical symptoms of anger outlined in earlier exercises. For example, the facilitator asks group members to clench their fists tightly. Next they are asked to relax their hands totally. This is a useful starting point in illustrating how muscular relaxation techniques may be used. Distribute handouts to interested parties and also (if available) suggest cassette tapes too. Emphasise that for relaxation training to be effective it is essential that the techniques are practised thoroughly *Before* 'difficult situations' for them to be truly effective *In* the situation. Another way of dealing with physical symptoms is to work out in the gym, thereby getting rid of the tension and energy associated with anger.

MANAGING ROLE PLAYS

Role plays can be a particularly effective way of helping clients learn anger management techniques. However, they require very careful management. Individuals participating in anger management groups can be potentially volatile. We recommend that role plays are used primarily at the later sessions of any anger management programme. As we have seen the later sessions tend to be focused primarily on the development and practice of anger management methods. Participants should be briefed as follows:

1 Make each participant's role clear.
2 Have a 'no physical contact' rule.
3 When the facilitator says 'stop', the action must end.

Initially it is best to keep role plays brief. One useful technique in lengthier role plays can be to 'stop' the action at key points to illustrate (and emphasise) key learning points. Role plays may also be helpfully videoed, which serves to give further opportunities for learning. In short, role plays are a powerful learning tool and we would strongly recommend their use, but with care.

SUMMARY

Anger management interventions involve a consideration of three psychological components to anger: arousal, behaviour and cognitions. Anger management treatment programmes target each of these areas. Organisational and planning issues in the political context of working within the criminal (or civil) justice system can be all important. Thus, it is important to establish how the intervention will 'fit in' with the goals of the organisation. A number of practical planning issues require careful consideration (see p. 129 for a list). Anger management programmes may be usefully structured to involve three stages: a general exploration of anger, the individual exploration of anger and anger management methods. We think that it is helpful to distinguish between process and content aims of individual sessions (with related objectives). This is because such an approach aids facilitators in ensuring that they give due consideration to the tasks required for a given exercise and also the dynamics of the relationships within the group. We strongly recommend that practitioners evaluate their work.

Chapter 10

What we know about sex offenders

THE RANGE OF BEHAVIOURS CLASSIFIED AS SEXUAL OFFENDING

Sexual practices have varied across cultures and throughout human history. Legal definitions of sex offending in the UK include a broad range of offences involving sexual victimisation of others and also acts which are 'victimless' in the sense that they may involve two consenting partners but still contravene societal norms. For example, acts of sadism between consenting adults are illegal in the UK. The age of consent for heterosexual intercourse is 16 years but is 18 years for homosexual intercourse. In this section we are concerned exclusively with sexual behaviour which victimises others in that they do not consent to the behaviour, or are unable to do so. Such offences can include both contact and non-contact offences.

Defined codes of sexual offending are clearly social constructs in that they have shown changing boundaries over time and between societies (Marshall *et al.*, 1990). It also seems clear that some behaviours are very widely seen as undesirable, and that some sexual behaviours are psychologically as well as socially dysfunctional. The *Diagnostic and Statistical Manual* of the American Psychiatric Association, version four (DSM-IV – American Psychiatric Association, 1994) refers to deviant sexual interests and behaviours as paraphilias (meaning a deviant interest) and categorises these with sexual dysfunctions within the broad heading of 'sexual and gender identity disorders'. This classification system lists eight main types of paraphilias plus a general catch-all class for other paraphilias. These are: exhibitionism (unwanted sexual displays); frotterism (sexual touching); sexual masochism (sexual pleasure through having pain inflicted on oneself); voyeurism (observing others' sexual activity or undressing); fetishism (sexual arousal to inanimate objects); paedophilia (sexual assaults on children by adults); sexual sadism (sexual pleasure through inflicting pain); and transvestic fetishism (dressing in clothes of the opposite sex). The catch-all classification of 'other paraphilias' includes scatologia (making obscene telephone calls), necrophilia (sexual interest in corpses) and zoophilia (sexual interest in animals) (ibid).

Rape is not included as a sexual disorder within DSM-IV, although some rapists would be classified within the sexual sadism group. Practitioners and researchers remain divided on the issue of whether rape should be classified as a sexual disorder. Some have argued that rape should be included as a separate paraphilic disorder (Abel *et al.*, 1977; Abel and Rouleau, 1990). Others have taken the view that rape should not be viewed as a sexual disorder at all but rather as a particular expression of male aggression towards women and children (Darke, 1990).

In this section we will focus on those who commit acts of sexual aggression against others, specifically rapists and offenders who molest children. These groups of offenders are frequently seen for assessment and treatment in forensic settings.

REPORTING RATES

Legally, sex offenders may be defined by one or more of the following factors: age difference between the offender and victim; the use of force, and the violation of kinship or close relationships. Thus, many of the paraphilias listed above may not be illegal and some sexual offences may have nothing to do with paraphilic interests. This is further complicated by the fact that many sex offenders may not be prosecuted under statutes and laws explicitly concerned with sexual behaviour. Making obscene telephone calls may often be sexually motivated but in the UK would be prosecuted under the Telecommunications Acts. This provides an illustration of how difficult it is to obtain an accurate estimate of the levels of sexual offending. In 1993 notifiable sex offences represented under 1 per cent of all notifiable crimes in England and Wales.

The trend in officially recorded sexual offences has been markedly different from other types of offending. Between 1963 and 1973 there was a steady and dramatic increase in convictions for sexual offences of around 25 per cent (Bottomley and Pease, 1986). This was followed by a steady decrease between 1973 and 1981, so that by 1983 the proportion of sexual offences was lower than that recorded in 1963. Since 1983 there has been a steady increase in sexual offences. These overall figures mask a dramatic rise in the level of reported rapes from 1,334 in 1983 to 4,589 in 1993. Again taking 1983 to 1993, indecent assaults have shown a parallel if less dramatic increase from 10,833 to 17,350. Gross indecency offences against children have also shown a dramatic rise from 513 to 1,280 (see Clark, 1993).

It remains unclear how far these changes reflect genuine changes in the levels of sexual offending, and how far they reflect an increased willingness to report such offences to the police.

VICTIM SURVEYS AND RANDOM SAMPLES

There is substantial evidence that the reported figures for sex offences dramatically underestimates the real level of such offending in society. The British Crime Survey in 1988 estimated that less than one-fifth of rapes and indecent assaults were reported to the police (Clark, 1993). Similarly it has been estimated that only about 10 per cent of those offences reported to the police would result in a conviction. The recorded rate for sexual offences being 'cleared up' by the police is higher than this since this category includes all cases where an individual is proceeded against, whether or not they are found guilty of an offence (see Bottomley and Pease, 1986).

Victim surveys may themselves underestimate true rates of offending. A number of studies now suggest that the use of aggression in sexual interactions is relatively common (Darke, 1986). For example, in a survey of 3,862 men and women college students in North America, 8 per cent of the women reported being physically coerced to have intercourse, whilst 3 per cent of the men admitted using physical force in this way (Koss *et al.*, 1985). A survey of a sample of young men in the US state of Oregon found that 13.5 per cent of respondents stated that they had engaged in sexually aggressive behaviour at some time in their lives. Perhaps the most alarming study is a survey of 930 adult women which found that 41 per cent reported sexual aggression to the extent of rape or attempted rape at least once in their lives (see Russell, 1975; 1984).

The extent to which men may be prepared to aggress sexually or rape has been studied. In a series of studies of college students in North America they were asked how likely it was that they might rape if they were assured of not being caught. The consistent findings were that 30–35 per cent reported that they would (see Malamuth and Check, 1983). Such studies can be criticised as being rather artificial experimental paradigms. It is also clear that individuals may respond very differently to hypothetical and real situations. Even allowing for such factors though, these studies do suggest a greater willingness to sexually aggress than has often been assumed by practitioners and researchers.

Similar survey studies have been conducted to look at rates of child molesting. For example, Finkelhor (1979; 1986) interviewed 530 women students and 266 men students, about sexual contacts with adults. He reported that 11 per cent of the women and 4 per cent of the men said they had experienced sexual contacts with adults before the age of 12. For the women, 37 per cent of these contacts were before the age of 9 and for men, 27 per cent were before the age of 10.

Using a somewhat wider definition of unwanted sexual contact, the Canadian National Survey reported on a random sample of 2,008 people. Of these 54 per cent of the women and 31 per cent of the men reported experiencing unwanted sexual advances at some point. The majority of these were reported as being before the age of 18 and most involved sexual touching, sexual assaults or attempted sexual assaults. The study also found that only 24 per cent of women and 11 per cent of men reported these contacts to anyone else (see Darke, 1990). Baker and Duncan (1985) with a sample of 2,019 people, found that 12 per cent of the women and 8 per cent of the men reported being sexually abused before the age of 16. In a survey of 1,244 British college students in which the researchers excluded offences such as exhibitionism and sexual contact with similar age peers; they reported that 21 per cent of the women and 7 per cent of the men said they had been sexually assaulted before the age of 18 (see Clark, 1993).

There are clearly wide variations in the levels of sexual offending reported by different researchers. Much of this variation it seems may be accounted for by variations in the definitions of offending and sexual aggression used. It is perhaps worth noting that none of these approaches have produced levels of offending as low as the officially notified rates of offending. Such studies as a whole tend to suggest that the rates of sexual offending are very much higher than the officially recorded figures for sexual offending. They would also suggest a relatively high propensity and willingness to use sexually aggressive behaviour particularly among men.

DESCRIPTIVE STUDIES

Those who assault adults

It has been argued that there are significant differences between rapists and other types of sexual offenders, leading some to suggest that rape is not primarily a sexual crime at all (e.g. Groth, 1979). Others such as Abel and Rouleau (1990) argue that in many cases rapists show very similar problems to other sexual offenders. Abel *et al.* (1988) in a group of 126 men who had raped adult women, found that 50 per cent reported onset of a deviant interest in rape before the age of 21. In clinical interviews they also found that many rapists reported recurrent, repetitive and compulsive urges to rape and fantasies about rape. These offenders reported a cycle of urges, attempts at control and then breakdown of control and offending. This, they argue, is similar to the pattern seen in other sex offenders. Additionally in Abel's sample of rapists 44 per cent had been involved in non-incestuous paedophilia, 28 per cent had an interest in exhibitionism, 24 per cent in incest, 18 per cent in voyeurism, 11 per cent in frottage and 10 per cent in sadism. This analysis has been criticised in that the sample used was a highly selected group sent for treatment from many parts of the United States. However, it does tend to call into question the view that all rape offences are an expression of violent rather than sexual behaviour.

Psychophysiological assessment has also tended to suggest that sexual motivations are important for at least some rapists. A comparison of sadists and rapists found that the rapists were aroused to portrayals of mutually consenting intercourse with adult partners, whereas sadists were not. Sadists were most aroused to portrayals of non-sexual physical assaults, which did not produce arousal in rapists (Abel *et al.*, 1981). Rapists appear to be distinct from other non-offending males in that they often fail to inhibit arousal to portrayals of violent sexual behaviours. Darke (1990) points out that the distinction between rapists and men who have not been convicted of rape is often far from clear cut, with high levels of variability within both groups. In addition she points out that the responses of 'non-offenders' to such portrayals can be easily disinhibited in the laboratory setting by portrayals which show the victim becoming sexually aroused (Darke, 1986; Malamuth and Check, 1983). Similar disinhibition can also be produced in the laboratory by provoca-tion (Yates *et al.*, 1984) and alcohol consumption (Barbaree *et al.*, 1983).

Suggestions that rape occurs due to a lack of access to consenting partners appears unfounded in the majority of cases. Groth and Burgess (1977) reported that most of the rapists they studied were involved in consenting adult relationships at the time of the offences. Similarly, the stereotype of the socially inadequate rapist appears wrong. Recent research has found no consistent social skills deficits in rapists which distinguish them from men not convicted of rape (Segal and Marshall, 1986; Stermac and Quinsey, 1986).

A fundamental flaw with this type of research into the characteristics of rapists has been the failure of researchers to establish clearly distinct groups of rapists and non-rapists on which to base their comparisons. The vast majority of studies have either relied on confidential self-reports from the men studied, or alternatively the absence of prior criminal convictions for rape. Given the low rates of reporting of sexual offences and the low success rate for prosecutions of such offences, this approach is wholly inadequate. One likely explanation of the large overlap between rapists and 'non-rapists' in many studies is simply that the latter group contains a proportion of unconvicted rapists (see Darke, 1986; 1990).

The use of force by rapists, in excess of that required to subdue the victim has been noted by many researchers, nearly all concerned with incarcerated groups (e.g. Amir, 1971; Groth and Burgess, 1977). Such aggression has been shown not to increase the sexual arousal of many offenders (Quinsey *et al.*, 1981). For those where violence was a factor in arousal this has been shown to be linked to a higher frequency and more violent offending (Abel *et al.*, 1978b). In non-rapists the woman's consent had a strong influence on sexual arousal. Portrayals of consenting sex produced responses of between 50 and 60 per cent of full arousal. More violent portrayals produced less arousal than two less violent portrayals. These differences became more pronounced on the second trial, suggesting that 'non offenders' were learning to inhibit arousal to such scenes. In rapists the results were less clear cut, with no significant reduction in arousal occurring in response to rape cues (Barbaree *et al.*, 1979; Baxter *et al.*, 1986).

The apparent variability in responding across groups of convicted offenders becomes easier to understand if rape is not viewed as a single offence in terms of motivation and offender characteristics. Knight and Prentky (1990) attempted to devise an empirically based and practically useful typology of rapists, building on earlier clinical typologies. They claim to be able to define nine subtypes of rapist with adequate reliability and validity:

1 Opportunistic (high social competence)
2 Opportunistic (low social competence)
3 Pervasively angry
4 Sexual sadistic (overt)
5 Sexual sadistic (muted)
6 Sexual (high social competence)
7 Sexual (low social competence)
8 Vindictive (low social competence)
9 Vindictive (moderate social competence)

(Knight and Prentky, 1990)

Whilst forensic clinicians disagree about the number and division of types, it does seem clear that this one legal category of offence can be committed for a variety of motives. Groth (1979) identified three types of rape offences: (1) anger rape; (2) power rape; and (3) sadistic rape, going on to assert that rape was primarily a violent offence where sexual behaviour was used as an expression of aggression. The typology by Knight and Prentky (1990) adds to this groups of rapists whose primary motivation is sexual.

Some studies have suggested that offenders show characteristic attitudes which distinguish them from non-offenders. In particular, it has been suggested that they show high levels of acceptance for what have been termed 'rape myths' (i.e. all women secretly want to be raped, victims really enjoy the experience of being raped). Acceptance of such beliefs has been found to be associated with self-reported sexual aggression in men not convicted of sexually aggressive offences (Koss *et al.*, 1985). It is unclear what this result actually means. It could also be argued that those who see rape myths as true are simply more willing to admit to sexually aggressive behaviours.

The majority of studies of incarcerated offenders have in fact found no differences in attitudes between rapists, other sex offenders or other males of similar social and economic backgrounds (Segal and Stermac, 1984). Other studies have found rapists to report more positive attitudes to women and less acceptance of rape myths than matched controls (Marshall *et al.*, 1984).

CHILD MOLESTERS

Howells (1979) compared what he termed non-familial child molesters with non-sexual offenders and incest offenders using a repertory grid technique. He found that child molesters and incest offenders saw adult relationships more in terms of dominance and submission. Adults also tended to be seen as overbearing by both these groups. This study gave some support to the notion that child molesters lack the social confidence to establish adult relationships. Behavioural studies of social skills have not detected any consistent pattern of deficits in child molesters (Stermac *et al.*, 1990). An emphasis on the behavioural components of social interactions alone may not be adequate to explain the complexity of social functioning problems, in that social functioning depends on the ability to interpret accurately social situations, as well as responding to them behaviourally. Some confirmation of this is offered in a study by Segal and Marshall (1986) in which child molesters were found to be significantly poorer at predicting and evaluating their own social performance in heterosexual social situations with adult women.

There is also some evidence that child molesters show deficits in social problem-solving skills involving adults and children. Offenders have been shown to be equally as good as non-offenders at recognising the presence of a problem, and at generating possible solutions. However, they showed a marked tendency to choose unacceptable solutions, and were poor at recognising likely negative outcomes (Barbaree *et al.*, 1988). Stermac *et al.* (1990) also report cognitive processing differences in respect of interpreting children's behaviours. In particular, child molesters perceived more benefit to the child from sexual behaviour, and attributed less responsibility and need for punishment of the offender than control subjects. Child molesters did seem able to pick up clear negative cues from children, such as a child becoming distressed. They differed most significantly where the child's responses were unclear or ambiguous.

INCEST OFFENDERS

Williams and Finkelhor (1990) point out that there has been a growing conviction among forensic clinicians that incest offenders are a distinct group from other child molesters. Until recently though, very little work had been concerned specifically with the characteristics of incest offenders. Early work tended to be based on clinical reviews, but little was done to validate such work empirically (see Butler, 1978; Cormier *et al.*, 1962; Herman, 1981; Lustig *et al.*, 1966). One exception to this was a study of incarcerated incest offenders (Gebhard *et al.*, 1965). However, incarcerated incest offenders are unrepresentative even of those incest offenders who are successfully prosecuted, since many do not receive custodial sentences.

In a review in 1990 Williams and Finkelhor reported that between 1978 and 1988 some twenty-nine empirical studies using adequate comparison groups were carried out, looking specifically at incest offenders. These studies were mainly small-scale and clinically based.

A popular hypothesis in the past has been that incest is transferred through the generations. This has not been at all well supported by the research. The highest rate of victimisation of incest offenders in any of the studies was 35 per cent (Baker, 1985) and the average across studies was reported to be around 20 per cent. The latter figure is not significantly higher than the levels of victimisation reported in some studies for the community as a whole (see Williams and Finkelhor, 1990). So, whilst it might be argued that such intergenerational transmission may be a factor in some individual cases, most commonly this is not the case.

Rates of physical abuse in the backgrounds of incest offenders were higher than the rates of sexual abuse. In three studies, rates of over 50 per cent were found. Incest offenders were not found to be distinct from physically abusive fathers (Lee, 1982) and non-familial sex offenders (Brandon, 1985) in the levels of physical abuse during their childhood.

The quality of relationship with their parents though, was found to be consistently poor, although evidence of separation is weaker (Williams and Finkelhor, 1990). Berkowitz (1983) used projective techniques to assess a group of incest offenders and reported significantly more themes of abandonment, powerlessness, maternal seduction and paternal rejection. Parker and Parker (1986) found that 50 per cent of incest offenders reported mistreatment by their father and 30 per cent by their mother.

The family backgrounds of incest offenders tended to show high levels of pathology in conflict resolution, trust, autonomy and intimacy (Saunders et al., 1986). Alcohol misuse was reported in 35 per cent of the families of origin (Baker, 1985). Parker (1984) reported that 35 per cent of offenders reported that their parents had a 'bad relationship' compared to a level of 13 per cent for a comparison group. These studies also found higher rates of incest against other family members in the offender's family background (Bennett, 1985; Brandon, 1985), giving some support for a modified version of an intergenerational transmission hypothesis.

A governmental review estimated that no more than 10 per cent of incest offenders showed any formal psychiatric disturbance (National Committee for the Prevention of Child Abuse, 1978). At least 25 per cent of incest offenders show no abnormality of personality (Scott and Stone, 1986; Langevin et al., 1985). A study by Langevin et al. (1985) did report that 47 per cent of incest offenders showed an elevated score on the psychopathic deviate score using a personality test (the Minnesota multiphasic personality inventory), a result which proved to be similar to a comparison group of non-familial child molesters. Lee (1982) found similarly elevated scores, but these did not differ significantly from a comparison group of fathers who physically abused their children. At best such results would suggest that incest offenders show a willingness to violate a broader range of social norms than most people. It is perhaps noteworthy though that most incest offenders do not have extensive histories of offending. This may suggest that their violation of norms is acted out in ways which do not come to the attention of the criminal justice system.

Quinn (1984) using an interpersonal behaviour survey found that a high level of dependency was the most important variable in discriminating between incest offenders and both 'clinical' and 'normal' comparison groups. This has been supported by other studies which have found very low levels of assertiveness, and also by clinical impressions (Langevin *et al.*, 1985). In contrast, Truesdell *et al.* (1986) found that 73 per cent of the mothers of incest victims had been physically abused, a rate similar to that found by Lee (1982) for fathers who were physically abusive to their children.

There appears to be some evidence that incest offenders are particularly prone to paranoid styles of thinking with some studies finding evidence of paranoid ideation (Langevin *et al.*, 1985; Lee, 1982; Fredrickson, 1981; Saunders *et al.*, 1986; Scott and Stone, 1986). It is unclear how far this may be a factor in the causation of offending and how far it is a reaction to the secrecy which surrounds such offending and the possible consequences of discovery.

The majority of researchers have found incest offenders to be of at least average intelligence on IQ tests (e.g. Maisch, 1972). Lee (1982), however, found that 10 per cent of a sample of incest offenders had IQs of less than 69, whereas in the comparison sample of physically abusive fathers none score below 69. Langevin *et al.* (1985) also found that on average their sample of incest offenders scored lower on IQ tests than either a community comparison group, or non-familial child molesters. Thus, while low intelligence is not a precondition for such offending it may be a significant factor in a minority of cases.

Early feminist theories suggested that incest offending was linked to the 'objectification' of children, particularly daughters, as a form of property. As such it was suggested that such offending would be particularly likely to occur in families where the father held rigid and stereotyped sex-role attitudes. Subsequent studies have failed to confirm this idea (Brandon, 1985).

The idea that incest offenders have poor marriages was not supported in a study by Parker and Parker (1986), who found no differences in this respect between incest offenders and matched groups of prisoners and outpatients. Thus, whilst levels of marital dysfunction were high, they were no higher than for other groups experiencing comparable social and psychological problems. No studies have yet tried to address the quality of the marital relationships prior to offending. Studies have, however, found significant differences in family functioning between families where incest has occurred and comparison families where it has not. Overall, the picture has been one where incestuous families show higher levels of social isolation, disorganisation, conflict and antagonism (Olson, 1982; Quinn, 1984; Saunders *et al.*, 1986). It is, though, difficult to estimate the extent to which such factors may have a role in causing or maintaining such offending, and how far they are effects of the offending.

Somewhat clearer is the evidence that incest offenders tend to show impaired empathy and bonding with their children (Parker, 1984; Parker and Parker, 1986). Incest offenders in these studies were more likely to avoid child care or nurturing activities (53 per cent compared to 24 per cent for non-offenders), and reported higher levels of discomfort about such activities. A higher proportion also reported being away from the household for all or part of the first three years of their victim's life (59 per cent compared to 14 per cent). Such findings would tend to contradict the notion that incest offenders are particularly emotionally close to their daughters.

Another consistent finding has been the presence of particular social skills deficits. In particular, incest offenders tend to report low levels of group activities and participation, with studies showing high levels of social introversion (Kirkland and Bauer, 1982; Langevin *et al.*, 1985; Parker, 1984; Scott and Stone, 1986; Strand, 1986).

RESEARCH INTO THE ROLE OF SEXUAL AROUSAL

Early pioneering work on sexual arousal in child molesters was undertaken by Freund (1967; 1981). These and later studies have produced quite consistent findings. As a group, non-familial child molesters who have assaulted girls show greater arousal to female children than non-offenders; they also tend to show arousal to adult women. Offenders who have molested non-familial male children show greater arousal to male children than non-offenders, whilst showing at least moderate levels of arousal to adult women and men. Non-offender groups show high levels of arousal to adults and a sharp drop in arousal to adolescents and children (Baxter *et al.*, 1984).

Barbaree and Marshall (1989) conducted a more detailed analysis of the patterns of sexual arousal shown by those who had offended against female children, incest offenders and matched non-offenders. They concluded that there were five distinct profile groupings in terms of sexual arousal patterns.

1 An 'adult' profile. With strong responses to adults of 20 years plus, moderate responses to the 16–18 years range and minimal responses to those under 15 years.
2 A 'teen–adult' profile. With strong responses to those of 13 years and over but weak responses below this.
3 A 'non-discriminating' profile. Showing moderate responses to all ages.
4 A 'child–adult' profile. With strong responses to those of 18 years plus and under 11 years and weak responses to the 12–14 years range.
5 A 'child' profile. With strong responses to the group under 11 years but only minimal responses to those of 13 years or over.

Just under 70 per cent of the non-offenders showed profile (1), with the remainder being evenly spread between (2) and (3). Of incest offenders 40 per cent showed an adult profile, 40 per cent were non-discriminating and most of the rest showed a teen–adult profile. Only one showed a child–adult profile. None of the non-offenders or incest offenders showed a pattern of responding exclusively to children. In contrast, non-familial child molesters showed very heterogeneous patterns of responding. The largest group, 35 per cent, showed the child-only profile. The remainder were quite evenly distributed across all of the other groups. It was clear that child molesters were not uniformly showing sexual arousal to children. Interestingly, those who showed the child and child–adult profiles had lower average intelligence (as measured by IQ tests), were of lower social and economic status and had used more violence in their offending. In terms of sexual arousal patterns, therefore, it seems clear that child molesters do not present as having a single pattern of problems.

Assessments specifically concerned with incest offenders' patterns of arousal to sexual stimuli have only recently begun. Marshall *et al.* (1986) found that on penile plethysmograph (PPG) measures, incest offenders showed a pattern of responding more similar to that of males not convicted of sexual offences than the patterns shown by non-familial child molesters. Whilst 19 per cent did show significant arousal to children, this was similar to the level for the 'normal' comparison group at 18 per cent. Incest offenders, though, were distinct in showing very low levels of arousal to adult women. The researchers concluded that incest offenders did not distinguish as much as non-offenders between pubescent and adult women, and in this respect appeared similar to non-familial child molesters. Among incest offenders and non-familial child molesters those with lower IQ scores were most likely to show deviant sexual arousal. Langevin *et al.* (1985) also reported that incest offenders reported more 'disgust' at sex with adult women than either non-offenders or non-familial child molesters. It is suggested that many incest offenders have conflicts about their adult sexual relationships which may result in arousal problems. This, even in the absence of significant arousal to children, may be important in leading to such offending.

CONCLUSIONS

The broad title of 'sex offenders' appears, from the research evidence, to be grossly misleading and potentially harmful. An enormous range of sexually aggressive behaviours is covered within a single legal category of offending. The area of sexual offending is also replete with loose thinking and the use of misleading terms. For example, child molesters may be described as 'homosexual' (e.g. Howells, 1979; Marshall *et al.*, 1990). This is misleading and often inaccurate in that some child molesters may be sexually active with adult women and aggress against boys, but have no sexual interest in adult men.

The research available suggests that groups of rapists and child molesters have characteristics which distinguish them from each other. Also, within these groups of offenders it seems clear that there are further distinctions. Rapists cannot convincingly be treated as a unitary group in terms of the development and nature of their offending. Early suggestions that rape is essentially a crime of violence rather than being sexually motivated seem to be wrong for many such offenders. At the very least we would argue that some such offences are motivated by sexual drives, whilst others are motivated purely by aggressive drives. The existing attempts to produce a valid typology of rape offenders appear to be a useful tool for assessment, treatment and future research.

Child molesters also appear to have clearly distinct characteristics. We would argue that the evidence suggests that for clinical and research purposes these groups are generally better seen as separate.

It is important when addressing the assessment and treatment of sexual offenders that there is clarity about exactly what offending has occurred. It is also important to look at the range of related offending and paraphilias.

SUMMARY

In this chapter we have reviewed some of the research into sex offending. We begin by discussing the research into the levels of such offending, as described by official figures and survey studies. The evidence from such studies suggests that sexual assaults are reported at a low rate, and that of those offences which are reported only a small proportion will result in a conviction. In turn only a proportion of those convicted will receive custodial sentences.

We then go on to discuss the research into those who assault adults and those who molest children. This includes consideration of the characteristics of convicted rapists and child molesters and how these compare with the general population of men. The majority of such studies have compared convicted rapists with groups of men not convicted of sexual offences. We suggest that this approach requires the caveat that, given the low rates of reporting, any random sample of men is likely to contain a number of undetected sex offenders.

We end with some general conclusions about sexual offending. Specifically we suggest that similar legal categories of offence can vary greatly, in terms of behaviour and also motivations.

Chapter 11

The assessment of sex offenders

INTRODUCTION

In this chapter we give guidance to practitioners on how to assess individuals who have committed sexual offences. We will also structure our discussion to cover ways of assessing the risk of sexual reoffending.

Practitioners in many branches of the criminal justice system, as well as those working in child care, will be well aware of a growing interest in sex offending. This seems to derive largely from an increased acknowledgment of historically high levels of sexual violence. The current Criminal Justice Act (1991) acknowledges this formally, and in recent years the Home Office in the United Kingdom has implemented a large-scale treatment programme for imprisoned sexual offenders. This is mirrored by developments in the health services, where a number of forensic healthcare services will have practitioners with expertise in working with such offenders.

In the wake of the Criminal Justice Act (1991) it seems likely that there will be continued growth in the amount of assessment and treatment work undertaken with sex offenders. This growth is likely to be most pronounced for the probation services, with obligations to provide input to offenders after release from prison and also non-custodial treatment programmes (McClurg, 1996).

Amidst this rapid expansion though, there remains a great deal of confusion about what constitutes good practice with such offenders. There is also considerable variation between and even within agencies in assessment practices. Below we outline a framework for conducting such assessments.

WHAT ARE THE FEATURES AND FUNCTIONS OF SEXUAL OFFENDING?

Sexual behaviour has a significant developmental component; the ways in which we express sexual drives are learned over many years. Accordingly any analysis of sexual offending needs to take a developmental perspective as well as looking at current behaviour. The main assumption of a cognitive–behavioural approach to sexual offenders is that their offending behaviours are learned and are triggered by external cues (e.g. someone they find sexually attractive) and internal cues (e.g. fantasies) (Marshall and Barbaree, 1990a).

A cognitive–behavioural assessment therefore aims to find out what these triggers to behaviour are. This will involve a detailed analysis of the events which occur prior to an offence, the behaviours involved in the offending and the events following the behaviour. This is often shorthanded by psychologists as an ABC analysis, standing for Antecedents, Behaviour and Consequences (O'Leary and Wilson, 1975). The cognitive–behavioural approach also requires consideration of cognitive elements such as a client's attitudes, beliefs, thoughts and fantasies, since these can influence behaviour.

PROBLEMS IN ASSESSING SEX OFFENDERS

There are a variety of characteristic problems involved in assessing sex offenders. These often include a lack of motivation to undergo assessment, embarrassment about discussing sexual behaviour and varying levels of denial about the offending. We discuss these in greater detail below.

Lack of motivation to undergo assessment

Complete denial

This most often seems to take the form of the offender asserting that they could not have committed the offence since they are not that type of person. Offenders denying in this way will refute the notion that they have any fantasies related to offending. They may often present as being extremely angry and outraged at such false accusations being made against them and can be very hostile to being assessed for treatment. One possibility here is that the client has not committed the offence(s). Practitioners should look at this question seriously in the light of the available evidence. However, often these individuals will have committed the offences but choose to deny it.

An alternative pattern is where the offender denies one or more offences on the grounds that they were not there at the times of the offences with which they have been charged. Such individuals will generally also deny any fantasies linked to sexually abusing others. In some cases they may concede the existence of these but question the relevance and significance, since they are being falsely accused (Salter, 1988).

Where there is convincing evidence that the person being assessed has committed the offence(s) the first task will be to challenge and, where possible, break down this denial. One way to do this is what is sometimes called 'motivational interviewing'. McGrath (1990) lists some guidelines for this type of interviewing. These include:

1 *Emphasising that assessment is a two-way process for the benefit of the offender.* This can be particularly important for many sex offenders who may have experienced a great deal of hostility and aggression due to their offending. This often leads sex offenders to refuse to engage in assessments or disclose any detail about their behaviour. This can sometimes be overcome by stressing the positive functions of such an assessment.

2 *Assumptive questioning.* For example, by asking about when the client committed the offence rather than if they committed the offence. Similarly, asking about when the client has sexual fantasies rather than if they do.

3 *Ignoring clearly untruthful answers.* Frequently in this context clients might say things which may be partly or completely untrue. When trying to increase a client's motivation to be assessed, it is generally counterproductive to challenge these statements directly. Equally, caution is needed in not seeming to agree with these. Effective approaches to this situation include simply continuing the current line of questioning as if that answer had not occurred. Or alternatively, switching to another line of questioning.

4 *Using strategies of successive approximation.* For example, getting offenders to concede that they committed a part of an offence. This will depend to a large extent on the starting point for the assessment. It can begin simply by getting the client to admit that they were in the area at the time or that they did speak to the victim. Other clients may be willing to concede that they touched a child. Such disclosures may allow the practitioner to try and elicit successively more honest and accurate accounts of the offence(s).

An assessment of a client who continues to deny any involvement in sexual offending at all, in the face of good evidence to the contrary, would generally raise concerns for practitioners, particularly when considering the offender's risk of reoffending. With those who admit even a very limited willingness to discuss aspects of their offending, progress towards reducing the risk of reoffending is more likely.

Partial denial

Whilst some clients will completely deny sexual offending, it is more common in most forensic settings to encounter some form of partial denial. This can take a variety of forms. Salter (1988) suggests that denial is not, as has often been assumed, a simple either/or situation between complete denial and complete admission. Instead she suggests that there are varying degrees and types of denial and that, for sex offenders, denial is a continuum involving several components. These suggested stages are outlined below:

1 *Admission with justification.* This is where the client admits their actions. For example, they might admit that they have abused several children. However, they justify this behaviour as acceptable or desirable. It has been suggested by some (e.g. Russell, 1975) that this is most frequently seen with rapists. It is also seen in the case of incest and non-familial child sexual abuse. This usually takes the form of arguing that the victim 'deserved' to be assaulted (e.g. a young woman walking alone at night). Or alternatively, that the victim benefited by the experience of being assaulted (e.g. the child was 'educated about sex' and this was good for them).
2 *Physical denial with or without family denial.* This might be where a client insists that they were not there when the offences occurred. Such denials may sometimes be supported by family members providing an alibi.
3 *Psychological denial.* This is where the client effectively says that they are not the type of person who could do this sort of thing, therefore they could not have done it.
4 *Minimising the extent of the behaviour.* Here the client accepts all or part of what they did but minimises it. For example, they might admit to touching a child inappropriately, but argue that this was purely accidental. Similarly, they may admit parts of their offending, but deny other aspects, for example, admitting indecent assault but denying rape.
5 *Denial of seriousness of behaviour and need for treatment.* This is where a client admits particular behaviours but argues that they were

not as serious as implied. For example, a rapist might argue that although what he did was clearly wrong the victim was not physically or psychologically injured by the assault.

6 *Denial of responsibility for behaviour.* This is where offenders admit the offending and acknowledge the seriousness of it, but externalise blame for their behaviour. A common example is that they were drunk at the time. If they had not got drunk they would not have offended in this way. Another example might be the suggestion that they were sexually frustrated because their wife would not have sex with them.

7 *Full admission with acceptance of responsibility and guilt.* This is where there is no denial but rather a full acceptance of responsibility for the offences.

Another form of denial sometimes seen is where the client accepts all or some of the previous offending, but denies that it is currently a problem due, for example, to a recent religious or moral conversion. Where the client uses this to suggest that there is no need for any further intervention, it can be seen as a different form of denial of responsibility. Salter (1988) suggests that in some cases such conversions will be motivated by a desire to avoid treatment. Genuine converts, she suggests, will not be resistant to treatment, but may benefit from their new-found faith during treatment. Certainly there is no evidence that religious conversion alone does anything to reduce the risk of sexual offending (Marshall and Barbaree, 1990a).

INITIAL INTERVIEWING

Effective interviews with sex offenders are dependent upon similar factors to any other type of interview with a client. Thus, the development of appropriate therapeutic rapport is important. Abel and Rouleau (1990) suggest that effective assessment interviews depend to a large extent on the skills and experience of the interviewer in dealing with this specific group of offenders. They suggest that the more evident it is that the practitioner has a good understanding of such offending then the more offenders will be willing to disclose. They also suggest that the duration of the therapeutic relationship and the degree of confidentiality being offered are critical in achieving accurate assessments of sex offenders. This view is reinforced by Kaplan (1985) who compared the levels of self-reported offending of two groups of sex offenders. One group were seen in a clinical mental health setting, the others were seen in a criminal justice setting. The latter group reported one-twentieth of the level of previous offending. Kaplan suggests that this difference was largely attributable to the fact that those in the clinical setting were offered complete confidentiality and would not be punished for disclosing previous offences. Abel *et al.* (1988) similarly stress the importance of such confidentiality in obtaining an accurate picture of the range, severity and frequency of an individual's offending. Whilst it is still possible to assess sex offenders without the very high levels of confidentiality advocated by some, it seems clear that such assessments will tend increasingly to underestimate true levels of offending as the level of confidentiality decreases.

Initial interviewing begins with a process of establishing an appropriate rapport with the offender and a framework for the assessment and treatment. In this context it is important that the practitioner makes explicit the limits to confidentiality. It is also sometimes helpful to outline the purpose of the assessment and what it is likely to involve. However unpleasant an individual's offending, we would argue that there is nothing to be gained in terms of assessment by taking an openly confrontational approach at this stage. Indeed, this can serve to further entrench an offender's denial and allow him to construe himself as a 'victim'.

Wherever possible practitioners should draw on any other available sources of information to confirm, or challenge, the offender's account. So, for example, we would suggest that offenders' accounts of being sexually or physically victimised themselves should whenever possible be confirmed by other sources.

Interviewing often most logically begins with an exploration of background factors. It is important to gather information about a client's family and developmental history. This would be followed by a detailed sexual history. In this, the practitioner would be trying to obtain as detailed and accurate an account as possible of an individual's previous sexual behaviours and experiences.

ANALYSING OFFENCES

From here the next step might be to ask about the offences. Where someone reports many types of offending it is often helpful to look at each type of offence using a similar framework, although it is often not necessary to analyse each and every offence. So, for example, if a client reports offences such as making obscene telephone calls, indecent exposure, indecent assault and rape, it is important to look at each type of offence in detail. However, where a client has many convictions for

Table 11.1 Interview schedule

Family background
Here the interview would focus on the client's family structure including their parents, siblings, foster or adoptive parents, time spent in children's homes or institutional care.

Developmental history
Does the client have any history of illness. Have they experienced any delays or problems in their development? This can be assessed by getting them to outline the main developmental milestones (e.g. start of puberty).

Sexual history
Here the practitioner should go through the client's sexual development including previous relationships/sexual experiences and activities engaged in.

Offending
A detailed history of offending is important in determining whether there has been any pattern of change in the client's offending. This would include interviewing about previous convictions, type of previous offences and any previous sentences.

Domestic situation
Current domestic situation should be covered. Does the client live alone or with others? Do they have easy access to young children? Do they have social or family support?

Previous assessments
Has the client undergone any previous assessment or treatment work. This should include dates, location and agencies involved wherever possible.

indecent exposure it is generally more appropriate to analyse a few incidents in detail. One approach to doing this is to use the Before–In–After (BIA) framework. This refers to the situation before an offence, whilst in the act of offending and after offending. This is functionally the same as using an Antecedents–Behaviour–Consequences framework, but is linguistically easier for the majority of clients to understand.

This can be done using a standard sequence of questioning for each of these stages concerned with the what? where? who with? when? and why? of the offending behaviour.

What? It is important to get an account of what actually happened prior to, during and after the offence(s). This can be facilitated by questions such as 'What were you doing one hour before your offence?' 'What did you do during the offence?' 'What did you do after the offence?'

Where? This will involve where a client commits their offences. Do they offend at home, or outside the home? Do they have favoured locations for offending (e.g. playgrounds)?

Who? Are there particular individuals that the client tends to offend against? Are their offences against adults or children? Are the assaults against one gender or both? Are there specific 'types' of individual targeted by the client (e.g. young girls wearing school uniforms)? It is also important to try and determine whether the client offended alone, or as part of a group, since this may have implications for any treatment work.

When? It is useful to get a picture of when the client offends and whether or not this is predictable. This can be important in developing an effective treatment approach.

Why? It is important to ask the client why they feel that the offence(s) happened. Most clients will have spent a great deal of time dwelling on their behaviour, and most will have some account of why they offend. These will include clients who say that society is wrong to outlaw sex with children when such behaviour is natural, and clients who will say their offending was due to sexual frustration. The amount of insight shown into their behaviour and its lack of acceptability will vary enormously. It is for this reason that it important to get the client's account as part of the assessment process.

OTHER ASSESSMENT METHODS

There are a range of approaches to the assessment of sex offenders. In general terms we would advocate the adoption of a broad-based and 'eclectic' approach to such assessments. This is because in the vast majority of cases sex offenders will show a range of psychological and behavioural problems linked to their offending. All of these will require careful assessment.

The use of a cognitive–behavioural framework in conducting such assessments can be highly effective. It aids practitioners by giving a clear framework within which to analyse what the offender says or does.

The cognitive–behavioural approach to the assessment of sex offenders is one of the applications of a more general synthesis between behavioural and cognitive psychology. The approach therefore makes several key assertions about the nature of behaviour in general, and offending in particular.

At its simplest this means that cognitive processes (e.g. thoughts, memories, fantasies) and the pleasure gained from particular behaviours are critical to the development and maintenance of sexual offending. The role of cognitive factors in behaviour has been increasingly recognised and in recent years clear theoretical frameworks have been developed to attempt to explain the links between thinking and behaviours. The best-known examples of this are probably cognitive models of depression (e.g. Beck, 1967). Similar cognitive models have been applied to sexual offenders (e.g. Murphy, 1990).

A cognitive–behavioural assessment of sex offenders serves more than one function for practitioners. We would suggest that these include:

1 Giving a clear analysis of target areas for intervention with an individual client.
2 Provision of structured information for evaluating the risk of re-offending by particular clients.
3 Allowing evaluation of the effects of treatment and also the ongoing development and refinement of intervention strategies.

As with other cognitive–behavioural assessments the approach is based on experimental approaches used by psychologists. So assessments can be seen as a logical process of generating credible hypotheses or ideas about offending behaviour and testing these empirically.

SELF-REPORT MEASURES

Interviews are the most frequently used and best-known means of obtaining self-reported information from clients. However, there are other methods which can be used in assessing sex offenders in this way. These include self-monitoring of behaviour and thoughts by the patient, usually in the form of structured diaries. Questionnaires can also be used and these provide another way to obtain self-report information.

Diaries

These can have some advantages over interviews. For example, they can serve to remind the offender of aspects or details of their thinking or behaviour which they may have forgotten about, or simply failed to attend to. Thus, it can highlight patterns in thinking and behaviour which are significant factors in the offences. Second, it provides an opportunity to challenge offenders to disclose more detail about areas such as sexual fantasies. Diaries can also give insights into factors which may maintain fantasies. Table 11.2 provides an example of this method.

The extracts in Table 11.2 give a brief example of a (well-kept) diary. Such diaries can be useful in that they may provide useful ideas about why an individual's problems occur. It may also suggest areas where further assessment is required. In particular, with this example it might be fruitful to explore the events which make this client angry. What happened? Who was involved? Where did the incident occur? How did they respond? Why were they angry? Similar analyses can also be conducted of the client's responses in terms of behaviours. In this case it can be seen that this individual masturbated in response to feeling angry. His favoured fantasy for masturbation was, in this example, young girls. Clients in general will find keeping such a diary difficult. It is therefore often helpful to go through such a diary format in detail. This may be done by getting the client to look back over the last few days and complete the entries with the help of the practitioner. Where clients are lacking in literacy skills, similar accounts can be tape recorded.

Perhaps, most importantly, such self-report diaries can give insight into internal psychological processes. Negative emotional states may often be precursors to relapses into a variety of compulsive behaviours (see Cummings et al., 1980). This also seems to be true for many sex offenders. Whilst much of this information may be obtainable through interviews, diaries can be a more effective means of gathering this information. They have the clear advantage that, if kept properly, they do not depend on a client's recall. This means that they will often provide a greater amount of detail than even the most motivated person can provide through interviews alone. In addition, by providing detailed and current information on an offender's thoughts and behaviours, they can allow more effective monitoring of the risk of reoffending.

Questionnaires

Questionnaires can be useful in conducting assessments because:

1 They allow the practitioner to compare a client's responses with a group of similar offenders.
2 They can allow comparison of offender's responses with those of non-offenders.
3 They can be used to compare a client's responses before and after treatment.

Table 11.2 Extracts from a client's self-report diary

Day	Mood (How strong 0 to 10)	Thoughts	Behaviour	How satisfying 0 to 10
Mon	Angry 8	Thinking about the little girls at work and how nice they are. How they always smile at me and don't put me down	Masturbated to the mail order catalogue. Looking at the school uniforms page	7
Tues	Depressed – row with wife 6	I'm useless. I can't keep anyone happy even me	Walked out. Went to the off licence and bought some cans of lager – drank them in the park – went home	1
Wed	Angry argument with my wife before I went to work 6	Why is she so demanding and aggressive to me all the time?	Stormed out to work	2
	Angry because the bus was late 4		Nothing – just waited for the bus	0
	Angry told off by my boss at work 10	He's just a bully. He doesn't know anything about my job. I should stand up to him. Then the same as Monday but all day at work this time	Accepted what my boss said and agreed with him	0
			After work – Went to the park on my way home to watch the children playing – felt a lot calmer after this	8

There are clear problems with using questionnaires with sex offenders. First, the fact that sex offenders will often have a wide variety of problems which may be linked to their offending means that there is no single questionnaire which can be used. Indeed, there is a large number and variety of these available. A second problem is that many of them are of very poor quality, and have not been shown to measure accurately what they claim to. Finally, as with all questionnaires, it is often very easy to see what the questionnaire is seeking to measure. As such, it is easy for a client to give socially acceptable answers, rather than responding in line with their own views.

One scale with wide application which we feel is useful is the multiphasic sex inventory (MSI) (Nichols and Molinder, 1984). This consists of 300 items which are marked true or false by the client. When scored, the MSI yields a number of scores relating to 'sexual deviance', 'atypical sexual behaviour', 'sexual dysfunction', 'sexual knowledge' and 'treatment attitudes'. The MSI also has the advantage of having four 'validity' scales, covering child molesting, rape, exhibitionism and incest. These are designed to assess how truthfully an individual is responding.

Whilst this test does have some value in informing a full assessment we would stress that it is not a substitute for such an assessment.

THE PENILE PLETHYSMOGRAPH (PPG)

This involves the presentation of stimuli to men whilst monitoring their erectile responses (Earls and Marshall, 1983). Stimuli for this assessment technique can take the form of still pictures, audio- or video-taped depictions.

The main value of PPG assessments are that they give evidence about an offender's responses to sexually explicit material which is based on their physiological responses rather than their self-report. If practitioners use self-report alone, then sex offenders may simply deny any inappropriate sexual arousal. Often they will do this for very logical reasons, such as the wish to avoid imprisonment or punishment. For this reason many researchers, particularly those in North America, have argued that the PPG provides a more objective way of assessing sexual arousal.

Penile plethysmography involves measuring the degree of penile tumescence in males in response to a range of stimuli. It is a non-invasive and non-painful procedure, although it may be confused by some clients with electrical aversion therapy. For this reason anyone undergoing such an assessment will need to have the procedure carefully explained. There are also a variety of technical and practical problems involved in this aspect of assessment, most of which are shared in common with other forms of physiological plethysmography (e.g. muscle plethysmography), and some which are specific to this particular measure. For this reason we would suggest that all such assessments need to be carried out and analysed by practitioners with the necessary specialist skills, training and experience.

In evaluating 'deviant' sexual arousal it is important to have accepted methods of measuring and evaluating this. Data from PPG assessments can be presented in a variety of forms, the simplest being the actual physical change. This is problematic since it makes no allowance for variations between individuals in sexual responding. It is more common to report data from PPG assessments as a percentage of full erectile response for that individual, thus correcting for such variation (Abel *et al.*, 1977). There are two widely accepted methods for doing this:

1 To measure the absolute levels of responding to particular stimuli, often expressed as a proportion of the full erectile response.
2 Calculating the relative level of response to deviant stimuli compared to non-deviant stimuli (see Abel *et al.*, 1978b; Marshall *et al.*, 1986).

Some authorities (for example, Quinsey and Earls, 1990) recommend both types of analysis as part of the assessment. They illustrate their case for this by giving the example of an individual who shows 50 per cent of his maximum arousal to an audio-taped account of an adult male having intercourse with a female child. The clinical implications of this may be quite different if it were accompanied by either high or low levels of arousal to adult consenting intercourse.

In either case the results of a PPG assessment will generally be presented in terms of what percentage of the full response was achieved for each type of stimulus material.

Carefully conducted PPG assessments have been shown to accord well with offending histories. Thus, offenders with a history of molesting young girls will tend to show high PPG arousal to young girls (Earls and Quinsey, 1985). PPG assessments have also been shown to illustrate patterns of deviant sexual interest even where the offender initially denies any such interest (Quinsey *et al.*, 1975). For this reason it is also important that the assessor discusses the results of the PPG assessment as soon as practicable after the assessment. This may serve to give the client more insight into their patterns of sexual arousal, or alternatively challenge misleading verbal self-reports.

Problems with PPG assessments

As an assessment technique PPGs are not infallible. It has been clearly shown that some offenders and non-offenders can exert considerable conscious control over their erectile responses (Quinsey and Chaplin, 1988). Whilst inappropriate sexual arousal can be an important aspect of offending this will not always be the case. Thus, some offenders seem to be able to control inappropriate arousal in a similar way to non-offenders, but choose not to exercise this control. Thus, a PPG assessment is valuable only as a part of a more extensive cognitive behavioural assessment. The research evidence does seem clear in suggesting that inappropriate sexual arousal is a major problem for very many sexual offenders, and is implicated in their offending (Quinsey and Earls, 1990). For all sexual offenders there will be other additional target areas for treatment also.

PPG assessments are essentially concerned with determining the category or categories of sexual partner and/or activities preferred by an offender. It is logical to assume that most offenders will act in accord with these preferences where possible. In reality though, sexual behaviour is often modulated by a range of factors other than preference, including opportunity, moral scruples, social resources and so on. Because of this all these factors are important in conducting an effective assessment.

The efficacy of PPG assessments also differs between offence types. Murphy and Barbaree (1988) reviewed the psychometric properties of PPG assessments. They concluded that for child molesters the procedure showed good levels of concurrence with the clients' offence histories. Compared to non-offenders child molesters also showed distinct and identifiable patterns of arousal. However, the picture for offenders who raped adults was much less clear cut. There was also a significant overlap between rape offenders and non-offenders. This gives some support for the idea that many rapists are not part of a clearly distinct pathological group (Darke, 1990). In the case of such offenders, other aspects of the cognitive–behavioural assessment are likely to be more productive than assessments of sexual arousal.

PPG assessments have also been shown to be open to distortion. Some offenders have been observed to fake responses by direct interference with the measuring device. Other methods such as tensing of the pelvic muscles or hyperventilation have been shown to influence PPG readings (Quinsey and Bergersen, 1976). In addition, it is clear that some individuals can exert a high degree of control over their erectile responses at will, or when instructed to do so (Wydra *et al.*, 1983). Direct attempts to interfere with the measuring devices can be dealt with using video monitoring, movement detectors and additional psychophysiological measures (in particular measures of muscle tension). It has though, proved more difficult to control for 'cognitive' strategies to control arousal. Geer and Fuhr (1976) demonstrated the effectiveness of using a relatively simple mental rehearsal task in reducing responses. These effects can be reduced by using particular systems of stimulus presentation, which measure the clients' ability to control arousal as well as their responses. The effects of such cognitive strategies, and the ability of some offenders to use these so well, should caution against an over-reliance on PPG assessments, particularly in the context of assessing risk of reoffending.

Another complication with PPG assessments is with the material presented. This seems to be particularly acute with video- and audio-taped stimulus material. Here an individual's labelling and interpretation of events portrayed may change over time, for example, from consenting to non-consenting intercourse. Also, even where the stimulus material is clearly non-consenting, care needs to be taken to remove any normal sexual cues which can cause arousal. Both of these processes can give misleading results on PPG assessments (Barbaree, 1990). This can largely be circumvented by the presentation of a second stimulus which omits the coercive aspects. A difference in levels of arousal can then be calculated.

Even though such techniques can be used, it remains very important to design stimulus materials very carefully. For example, a large number of non-offending males will become aroused to rape scenes where the victim is shown to become sexually aroused. Where this is not the case, the majority of non-offenders will show greatly suppressed arousal relative to consenting intercourse (Malamuth and Check, 1980). For assessment purposes it is therefore important, in this example, to remove suggestions of the victim becoming aroused in the stimulus material.

In addition, it may be the case that the same level of arousal to a given stimulus may have different clinical implications for two clients. So where one client shows 50 per cent arousal to consenting sexual intercourse and no arousal to sadism, the implications will be very different from a client who shows 50 per cent arousal to consenting intercourse and 100 per cent arousal to sadism.

Finally, it is worth noting that there are considerable ethical problems with the production of stimulus materials for PPG assessments. By definition those being assessed will become most aroused to activities which are illegal and severely damaging to others. As such, production of video or pictorial stimuli of this type would be both illegal and unethical. Some treatment centres have circumvented this by using illegal pornography seized by the police or law enforcement agencies. However, again we would argue that this effectively further victimises those who have been involved in the production of such material. For this reason alone we would see this approach as unethical. The vast majority of UK treatment centres have adopted an approach of using audio-taped descriptions of particular deviant sexual interests. This has the advantage that it does not further victimise anyone. In addition, it allows the stimulus material to be tailored specifically for each offender, giving more effective assessments.

WRITING ASSESSMENT REPORTS

A full cognitive–behavioural assessment of a sexual offender will produce a great deal of information. It is therefore important that the practitioner thinks carefully about the requirements of the target audience. Clear distinction between opinions and factual information is also important.

For our purposes we will assume that the report is structured to help inform treatment intervention decisions. Hence a full report will need to include information on:

1 The client's level of denial before, during and after the completion of the assessment.
2 An assessment of any aspects of development which appear to be related to subsequent offending.
3 A detailed analysis of offending behaviours. This should cover any patterns of behaviour in terms of the development of these. It should also include an analysis of when and where the client offends and whom the client offends against. The assessment report should also give details of the thoughts, fantasies, emotions and behaviours which the client reports before, during and after offending.
4 A summary of any questionnaire information collected in terms of what this tells us about the client's patterns of offending.
5 A summary (where applicable) of any PPG assessment, again in terms of what it tells us about the client's patterns of offending.

SUMMARY

In this chapter we have covered the assessment of sex offenders. We advocate a broad-based and eclectic approach to such assessments, on the basis that many sexual offenders will have multiple problems which may be linked to their offending. Thus, areas such as social skills, substance abuse and anger management may all require assessment. Within this broad eclectic framework, the use of a cognitive–behavioural model with sex offenders has proven to be an effective approach. It has the advantage of structuring the assessment in a way which guides later treatment work. It also provides a logically coherent framework for assessing the risk of reoffending.

Where possible, assessments of sex offenders should involve more than one assessment method. The most frequently used method is the interview. Self-report diaries and questionnaires can also be of value. Physiological measures of arousal can also be a useful aid in assessing inappropriate sexual arousal for some offenders. Such measures are achieved by means of a penile plethysmograph (PPG). In common with other physiological measures this method requires very careful use and interpretation.

An assessment of sex offenders within a cognitive–behavioural framework will structure information about offenders in a way which will aid practitioners in making effective assessments of treatment needs and of the risk of reoffending.

Chapter 12

The treatment of sex offenders

In this chapter we begin with a brief introduction to sex offender treatment work. Then we move on to the main focus of the chapter, giving a detailed examination of practice issues including planning issues, exercise content and processes, group dynamics, the management of group exercises, evaluation issues and an examination of difficulties and suggested solutions.

SEX OFFENDER TREATMENT WORK – HOW TO DO IT

In this section we will cover organisational, selection, planning, debriefing and evaluation issues. Then we will outline a selection of exercises and details of how they may be facilitated. Finally, we examine a number of common difficulties which may arise in undertaking such work. Our primary focus in this final section is in giving pointers to assist practitioners in anticipating and ameliorating difficulties to help enhance the treatment programme.

INDIVIDUAL VERSUS GROUP-BASED INTERVENTIONS

Wherever possible, interventions aimed at reducing sexual offending are better conducted using a group-based approach. There are several reasons for this. Particularly important among these are:

1 That a group-based approach serves to challenge and break down the secrecy which is often inherent in sexual offending.
2 It makes it clear to offenders that others have similar problems controlling their sexual behaviour, and are motivated to improve this control.

3 In many cases sex offenders can be very effective at identifying and challenging distorted or inaccurate accounts of each other's offending.
4 Offenders are often best placed to suggest credible alternative and coping behaviours.

There are, though, cases where group-based approaches are not initially suitable. For example, offenders suffering from a psychiatric disorder involving delusional beliefs or hallucinations are unlikely to benefit until these are dealt with first.

Individuals with learning disabilities can benefit from group interventions. These may need to be tailored specifically to their needs. In general terms the approach is similar. Concepts are likely to need simplification and the pace of the group is likely to be much slower. Where such provision is not available individual work may be required.

ORGANISATIONAL AND PLANNING ISSUES

As with all types of intervention work it is important to have an awareness of the political context in which practitioners work. Intervention work with sex offenders does not occur in a social vacuum. In criminal justice systems practitioners are likely to be acutely aware of the increasingly highly politicised nature of their work at a number of levels. In practice, this awareness will be helpful in informing the judgements about how the work fits into the agency or organisational setting. We would not wish to be overly prescriptive about this area. However, it is potentially important because if full consideration is not given to such basic organisational issues, the whole programme may be undermined. There are a number of questions which may be helpful at this initial stage. Who else other than the identified client will be affected by the client's participation? Who else is working with the client? What, if any, other work is being done? Who will need to be informed of the work? How does the work fit into the priorities of the organisation or agency? What level of management support will there be?

Once it is agreed and understood precisely how the group work will 'fit into' the organisational context a number of very practical organisational arrangements need to be clear. A brief checklist is given below.

Checklist for planning sex offender groupwork: practical resources and arrangements

1 Locate an appropriate venue.
2 Be clear about how long sessions will be and when the group will meet.

3 Establish who the group facilitators will be.

4 Decide upon what is going to be included in the programme.

5 Arrange time to review precisely how the programme will be implemented.

6 Establish how and when the selection of candidates will take place.

7 Ensure that a maximum of ten people are on the group.

8 Agree how the group will be evaluated.

9 Brainstorm possible practical problems and generate a range of possible solutions.

Considerations in the selection of an appropriate venue would include ensuring that there is an adequate level of privacy, sufficient space, that the participants will be comfortable and that there is easy access to the venue.

The spacing of the sessions is important. Facilitator and client availability are primary considerations here. Also, in terms of the groupwork the spacing of sessions will have an impact. Broadly, the greater the interval between sessions, the greater the opportunity for clients to undertake 'homework assignments', which are important. The closer the sessions are together, the easier it is to maintain and develop a sense of group cohesion. A rate of two to three sessions per week may be about the right balance for session spacing in view of these two biases.

It is probably best to have two facilitators when undertaking sex offender groupwork. This is because it is demanding work which requires a high degree of sensitivity and awareness to the needs of participants. For these reasons it is also preferable to have consistency in facilitators. This does not mean that an entire programme must be facilitated by the same two people. However, there should be a small team of no more than three or four facilitators.

When deciding upon a programme of sex offender groupwork, it is worthwhile trying to look at as many examples as possible. We strongly recommend that programmes should include exercises to help clients deal with their sexually related arousal, behavioural and cognitive appraisals. Above all, ensure that the exercises you select are relevant and focused to the needs of the individuals on the group.

Setting aside time to talk through the logistics of precisely how each exercise will be facilitated is very important indeed. There are usually many different ways in which exercises may be run. Much of the finer detail is probably best left to the planning and debriefing meetings between group sessions.

It is absolutely essential that an effective method of selection is used.

In the case of sexual offenders we strongly recommend that a full assessment is carried out prior to any intervention. A possible framework for such an assessment is given in the previous chapter. All prospective candidates should be assessed individually and in depth. This is critical because a treatment intervention which is inappropriately applied may increase the risk of subsequent sexual offending. Those referred for sex offender groupwork should:

1 Acknowledge that their sexual offending is unacceptable.
2 Express a willingness to talk about their sexual offending difficulties in front of others with similar difficulties.
3 Express a desire to change and further develop the control they have over their sexual behaviour.
4 Express a willingness, and demonstrate their ability, to contribute constructively to a group respecting the rights of others.

In addition to the guidelines given above, just as with any groupwork intervention, when selecting candidates it is worth considering the 'mix' of participants. There needs to be a balance between those who are confident about speaking in a group and those who are less socially competent. It has also been suggested (e.g. Beckett, 1994) that it is important to have a mix of types of offenders, otherwise they will fail to identify and challenge each other's cognitive distortions. Whilst there may be some truth in this, we would suggest that the case for this has often been overstated. Effective facilitation can circumvent such a tendency.

It is a good idea always to ask prospective candidates if they anticipate any difficulties in attendance. As a general approach it is useful to go through your interview structure with the client as part of a matching process. In other words, explain what is available, emphasise that you are assessing its suitability for the client as much as his suitability for it. Thus, the interview is concluded by making a decision about the suitability of the groupwork in meeting the client's needs and the suitability for the groupwork being offered.

Generally, it is understood in the groupwork literature that between six and twelve candidates for groupwork intervention is about right as an environment to ensure the best opportunity of a group functioning effectively (e.g Brown, 1989). For this type of group, ten should be seen as a maximum limit. This is because of the intensity of the work.

The effective evaluation of individual and groupwork interventions with sex offenders is notoriously difficult (Crighton, 1995; Crighton and Towl, 1995). However, it should be part of the programme to build in an evaluation. Evaluation may be conducted in a number of ways. These can range from measuring how much participants enjoyed the group, through to evaluation of reoffending. The latter is, we suggest, the most significant aspect of evaluation for sex offenders. It is very difficult to measure true rates of reoffending due to factors such as the low rates of reporting of sexual crimes. However, these difficulties can and have been largely overcome or at least ameliorated by some treatment centres (e.g. Marshall and Barbaree, 1990b).

THE FIRST SESSION

As a general rule in groupwork the first session is the most anxiety provoking for all concerned. First impressions count. Both facilitators and clients benefit from the social investment involved in the selection process. Familiar faces take the edge off anxieties. Information gained during the selection interview may form the basis of informal interaction (and dialogue) whilst the group is assembling.

An essential task in the first session is the spelling out of the group rules. The principles include the facilitators needing to make it clear precisely what they expect of the clients. Equally, it is important to spell out what service is on offer. When making explicit what is 'on offer' it is important to include an overview of the groupwork and its purpose.

The course is divided into three parts:

1 Understanding sex offending.
2 An individual examination of offending behaviour.
3 Methods of preventing offending.

Each of these requires a high degree of participation from the group. The aim of the course is to help clients increase their control over their sexual behaviour. The facilitators need to make a statement of their commitment to the work. They also need to stress the individual responsibility of each group member for what they get out of the group. The inclusion of a cliché such as 'You will get as much out of this group as you put in' is generally well received. It serves to structure expectations in the direction of a high degree of participation by clients.

Group rules must include basic logistics, e.g. the number (and times) of sessions and also the venue. Stress the need for punctuality – this cuts both ways – facilitators will need to arrive on time too. There is little enough time. Make a statement about the fact that all clients have been selected because of their suitability and commitment to the work. The whole group benefits from each individual's contribution. It is critical at this stage to outline the boundaries of confidentiality within (and without) the group. The expectation is (as agreed at the selection interviews) that participants will attend *all* sessions. However, it is recognised that within some environments, this is sometimes not possible for good reasons. If anyone is unable to attend a session, it is essential that they discuss this with the facilitators beforehand. It is not acceptable for anyone to miss a session without having informed the facilitators. Basic democratic principles of interaction will also need to be spelt out, e.g. everyone is entitled to express their opinions and be listened to. It is useful to emphasise the benefits of working as a group, e.g. the benefits of joint understanding and problem solving. It is also important to spell out that the facilitators will not tolerate any derogatory language, abuse or threats directed towards others.

It is very important that facilitators make it clear from the outset that the bulk of the behavioural and cognitive control methods outlined and suggested during the group are taken from a number of similar previous groups. The facilitators cannot offer 'solutions' but rather 'suggestions' which others with similar difficulties have found useful.

The facilitators sometimes may find it helpful to say something about how, within the groups, not all suggestions of control methods will be effective for everyone, but past experience has shown that everyone will find some suggestions of use.

During the facilitation of the first session it is especially important to encourage all to participate. This does not mean that everyone has to say something. Verbal contributions provide a helpful indication of someone's level of involvement in the group but so do non-verbal responses, e.g. smiles and nods of agreement or acknowledgement. However, facilitators should ensure that everyone is given the opportunity to ask questions or clarify any points. It is important to try to ensure that everyone who appears to want to contribute verbally has the opportunity to do so.

The session should conclude by thanking the group for their attention/ participation.

EXERCISES FOR SEX OFFENDER GROUPWORK

This selection of groupwork exercises fall under three headings.

1 Understanding sex offending.
2 Individual examination of offending.
3 Preventing offending.

Each exercise in each of the sections begins with a 'content aim' and 'content objectives' followed by a 'process aim' and 'process objectives'.

The content aim and objectives provide the practitioner with guidelines to work through the structure of a given exercise. The content aim is a general statement of what information needs to be conveyed during the exercise. The content objectives guide the reader in a more detailed consideration of how to meet the content aim.

The process aim and objectives are principles for the practitioner to take account of and work towards during each exercise. The process aim is a general statement of what underlying principle to work at in each exercise. The process objectives specify practical ways of achieving the process aim.

So, in sum, the content aim and objectives give the exercises some basic structure. The process aim and objectives provide principles to link into group discussion.

UNDERSTANDING SEX OFFENDING

Exercises I, II and III are best facilitated using a flipchart, a selection of coloured felt tip pens and adhesive putty. It is helpful to keep all the materials generated in these exercises in full view throughout the sessions. Such materials may be referred back to during subsequent sessions, especially to illustrate learning points and remind the group of the ground covered. Facilitators may use these materials as cues to explore points raised in more detail or simply to clarify particular points.

Exercise I

Content aim

To understand 'sex offending'.

Content objectives

1 To get an indication of what *situations* group members associate with high potential for committing sex offences.
2 To get an indication of what *thoughts* group members associate with a loss of self control over their sexual behaviour.
3 To get an indication of what *feelings* group members associate with a loss of self control over their sexual behaviour.

Process aim

To elicit a sense of group cohesion and individual involvement.

Process objectives

1 To encourage as many responses as possible at each stage of the exercise.
2 To point out commonalities and acknowledge individual differences in contributions elicited.

Exercise brief

The words **SEX OFFENDING** are written at the head of a sheet of paper on a flipchart.

1 Group members are asked to say what *situations* they associate with their offending. Typical responses include: pubs, nightclubs, playgrounds and at home.
2 Group members are asked to say what *thoughts* they associate with sex offending. Typical responses include: 'She's asking for it', 'I'll teach him/her about sex', 'The tart', 'It won't do her any harm', 'I'll teach her to be so stuck up' and 'Children are interested in sex, they enjoy it'.
3 Group members are asked to say what *feelings* they associate with sex offending. Typical responses include: sexual frustration, hatred, tension and jealousy.

Exercise II

Content aim

To outline a model of sex offending.

Content objectives

1 To indicate that susceptibility to a loss of control over sexual behaviour fluctuates over time.
2 To indicate that we may be aware that our underlying levels of emotion may increase over the course of a sequence of events.
3 To indicate that certain events may act as 'triggers' to sexual offending.

Process aim

To get the group to identify with the model.

Process objective

To use participants' contributions from earlier exercises to illustrate the model.

Exercise brief

A model of sexual offending is outlined to the group in terms of the steps leading up to offending. The framework below is based on one described by Finkelhor (1984). However, it may be helpful to make it clear that this model is based on what other groups of offenders have said, rather than being simply 'made up' by the facilitators.

Step 1. Wanting to offend.
Step 2. Giving yourself permission to offend.
Step 3. Putting yourself in a position to offend.
Step 4. Overcoming victim resistance.

Each of these steps can be seen as part of a pattern leading up to particular behaviours. Step 1 involves the initial desire to offend, such as becoming aroused by fantasising about or seeing a potential victim.

Step 2 will involve the individual telling themselves that it is okay to do what they want to do. This will often involve some of the thoughts about sex offending which may have been elicited during Exercise I. For example, the belief that the behaviour 'will not do any harm to the victim'.

Step 3 will involve offenders putting themselves in a position where it is possible for them to offend, for example, by being out late at night, or babysitting alone.

Step 4 involves using various methods to overcome the victim; these can include physical force, but may also involve threats or bribes.

The facilitator links the model to the general and/or specific comments about sexual offending already elicited from group members.

Exercise III

Content aim

To convey the possible effects of sexual offending on victims.

Content objective

To encourage the group to consider the physical and psychological damage which can be caused by their offending.

Process aim

To increase empathy with victims of sexual offences.

Process objectives

1 To encourage the exploration of physical damage caused by sexual offending.
2 To encourage the exploration of the psychological damage done by sexual offending.

Exercise brief

Group members are divided into pairs and given written accounts from victims of sexual assaults to read through. Examples of such accounts are contained in the prison service treatment programme (HM Prison Service, 1994). Each pair should then spend time discussing and listing the main *feelings* and *effects* reported by victims of sexual assaults. These are then fed back to and discussed within the whole group.

This exercise can also be run using videotaped accounts from victims of assaults. Several treatment centres in the UK have used material from televised documentaries, drama and discussion programmes. If carefully chosen, these can act as very powerful catalysts for eliciting the feelings and effects of victims of sexual assaults.

Facilitators should bring out the main points on a flip chart/blackboard about the feelings and damaging effects on the victims of sexual assaults. These should include at least:

- Feelings of powerlessness.
- Physical injury.
- Long-term fears.
- Depression in later life.
- Self-injury in later life.
- Low self-esteem.
- Later sexual/relationship problems.

INDIVIDUAL EXAMINATION OF SEX OFFENDING

During the 'individual examination of offending' exercises, the dominant activity from the facilitators' viewpoint is in establishing a detailed individual account of each group member's pattern of offending.

Exercise IV

Content aim

To elicit detailed individual accounts of offending.

Content objectives

1 To break down accounts into a number of discrete (although directly linked) events.
2 To clarify what, if anything, happened between identified events.
3 To encourage the group to ask questions of and constructively challenge each individual account given.

Process aim

To demonstrate that sexual offending tends to be part of a largely predictable sequence of 'steps', with the client making decisions with each step.

Process objective

To encourage an awareness of the links between the sequences of behaviours and events which result in sexual offending.

Exercise brief

1 Each group member is asked to give a brief individual account of their offences. It is important to give some structure to such accounts in terms of suggested subheadings. The four-step model described in Exercise II provides a good framework for this. Key issues are identified and written up on the blackboard/flipchart under the headings of: (i) thinking about offending, (ii) excuses; (iii) making opportunities; and (iv) overcoming the victim.

It is particularly important that facilitators ensure that they have a sufficient understanding of the event outlined. This is important because such information is critical in making a full assessment of each individual's difficulties.

2 Once each group member's account is up on the blackboard/flipchart they are analysed by the group. The facilitator initiates the analysis for each account by asking the group 'At what point was there no turning back?' 'Why was this?' Disagreements or differences of opinion about the answers to such questions are examined further in discussion. In terms of structuring the discussion the facilitator cannot go far wrong (!) if they keep the discussion within the labels – the background, situation, thoughts, feelings and consequences. Although at this stage it is probably not necessary to 'fit' reported experiences directly with these labels, it is important to have a general idea of the significance and meaning of events for individual group members. The facilitator must clarify their understanding of the reasons 'behind' individual group members' answers.

Exercise V

Content aim

To outline the BIA model of sex offending.

Content objectives

1 To link the BIA model to the 'steps' model outlined in Exercise II.
2 To illustrate the BIA model using examples from accounts already elicited from individual group members.

Process aim

To encourage an understanding of a straightforward framework for the subsequent generation of self-control strategies.

Process objectives

1 To emphasise the importance of self-awareness in anticipating potentially difficult situations at the *Before* stage.
2 To emphasise the need to have a set of strategies to use *In* situations where there is a significantly increased risk of reoffending.

3 To emphasise the need for self-reflection, self-criticism and/or self-praise at the *After* stage.

Exercise brief

Introduce the BIA model of offending. It is essential that when introducing the BIA model, examples are used to illustrate the three stages. Where possible and appropriate, use examples previously given by group members. Explain that:

1 *Before* involves self-awareness, the anticipation of events and practice or rehearsal of self-control skills, awareness of decision making, avoiding high-risk situations.
2 *In* involves the awareness that things may be getting out of hand and using certain strategies and skills to cope with the situation.
3 *After* involves self-reflection, self-criticism and/or self-praise.

Distribute handouts on BIA. Encourage discussion in exploring the BIA model in terms of the individual accounts given by the group members. Link BIA to the earlier used 'steps' model of the manifestation of sexual offending (see Exercise II).

Exercise VI

Content aim

To promote an understanding of the effects of beliefs on behaviour.

Content objectives

1 To encourage group members to list a number of relevant beliefs.
2 To encourage group members to make explicit the links between their beliefs and behaviour.
3 To suggest possible links between identified beliefs and behaviour.

Process aim

To develop an awareness that beliefs are not 'given' facts and that they may be subject to scrutiny and reflection in the light of their influence on behaviour.

Process objectives

1 To encourage critical self-reflection on the link between beliefs and behaviour.
2 To encourage the exploration of self-serving beliefs.
3 To emphasise the consequences of holding particular beliefs.

Exercise brief

Ask group members to share their beliefs which are associated with their offending. Always give examples, e.g. 'If a young woman is out alone late at night she's asking for it'. Get group members to identify core beliefs which they use to give themselves permission to offend.

You may wish to talk through an example to illustrate the link between beliefs and behaviour. For example, by getting the group to generate as many reasons as possible to excuse speeding in a car. These examples can then be linked back to the main theme of the session, namely that beliefs can be used to give ourselves permission to behave in ways which are wrong (i.e. ideas can be self-serving).

In the group discussion the facilitators should encourage the exploration of beliefs. However it is critically important *not* to remain neutral about particular beliefs and to challenge certain beliefs (e.g. the self-serving idea that young children are sexually curious and therefore benefit from sexual intercourse).

Methods for doing this effectively can be drawn from other types of cognitive intervention techniques developed to address a wide range of behavioural and psychological difficulties (e.g. Beck, 1991; Meichenbaum, 1977).

It is important here not simply to argue or disagree with group members. The approach instead would involve:

1 Getting offenders to identify the thoughts which are associated with their offending.
2 Checking the feelings associated with the statements, for example by asking ' When you think that how does it make you feel?'
3 Leaving the validity of the statement open and exploring the evidence that the offender has to support that belief.
4 Exploring and challenging this evidence by using real information about the nature and effects of sexual assaults.

This is perhaps best explained using a case example.

Danny

Danny was admitted to a secure health service hospital having sexually assaulted both his daughters between the ages of 6 and 12 years. He argued that they were sexually curious and had enjoyed intercourse with him. His evidence to support these beliefs was that the girls had been affectionate towards him and became upset and distressed when he was finally arrested. That they did not immediately report him provided him with support for his distorted view of reality. So did the fact that they did not cry out or fight him. In addition, he argued that they had to have sex eventually and it was better for them to be educated by him.

Here the practitioner might work on the objective information relating to Danny's supporting evidence, rather than the main belief. So, for example, it is clearly true that most young children will be affectionate towards their parents. Most will never have sex with their parents, so this is unlikely to be the motivation for their affection. In this case Danny's daughters also became much less affectionate towards him after he had assaulted them.

Danny's idea that because the girls had not cried out and fought him they had enjoyed the sexual assaults was most easily challenged by the medical evidence. As is often the case, the victims in this case have suffered severe injuries in the form of vaginal and anal tearing, and related haemorrhaging and infections. This had led to severe pain in urinating and defecating. This was tested by getting Danny to rate how enjoyable he would rate each of these experiences and how likely he thought it was that his daughters had enjoyed going through these experiences. Would his daughters really think he had been affectionate to them?

It is also possible to use of role play techniques in this context (e.g. Abel *et al.*, 1978a). This essentially involves the use of role-reversal techniques where the practitioner will role play the offender and the offender is required to role play the professional trying to change the offender's rationalisations and distorted thinking. Whilst such techniques can act as powerful therapeutic tools, they appear to depend to a very large extent on the confidence and knowledge of the practitioner. To use such methods a practitioner needs to have a very good knowledge of the types of distorted thinking shown by sex offenders and be able to role play these convincingly. They also need to be able to make the links between such exercises and the offender's own ways of thinking. We would advise great caution in using this technique.

PREVENTING OFFENDING

Exercise VII

Content aim

To get a detailed account of an individual's offending using the BIA model.

Content objectives

1 To encourage group members to apply the BIA model to examples of their offending.
2 To encourage group members to challenge self-serving beliefs in each other's accounts of offending.
3 To encourage group members to identify seemingly irrelevant decisions in each other's accounts of offending.

Process aim

To provide group members with a straightforward conceptual framework to help them explore and understand their offending.

Process objective

To encourage group members to give an accurate account of their own offending.

Exercise brief

Reintroduce the BIA model stressing the importance of self-awareness and the anticipation of difficult situations. In this exercise the idea is to focus on the situational aspects of individual accounts given.

Offenders should then talk through their offending for the group. This will involve them talking through examples of each type of offence they have committed. During this the group should constructively challenge any efforts by the individual to minimise their behaviour, or blame others.

This is often a stressful exercise for all group members. Some will find it harder than others to talk about their offending to the whole group. It is important therefore that the facilitators ensure that the group remains constructive in their challenging.

Exercise VIII

Content aim

To demonstrate the applicability of 'self-talk' strategies in controlling behaviour.

Content objectives

1 To encourage group members to list a number of self-talk statements which may be of use before and in situations where they are at risk of offending.
2 To suggest self-talk statements which may be of use to particular individuals in the group.

Process aim

To get group members to acknowledge and apply self-talk strategies in negotiating their way out of potentially 'high-risk' situations.

Process objectives

1 To ask group members to recount what they have said to themselves in situations where they did not offend.
2 To ask group members to recount what they have said to themselves in cases where they did offend.
3 To emphasise the major role of 'self-talk' in critical situations.

Exercise brief

Introduce the notion of 'cognitive self-talk techniques'. Rework examples given in the earlier exercises (e.g. Exercise III) with the group. Scrutinise the examples in terms of possible 'self-talk' strategies to help each other deal more successfully with such situations. In particular, group members should try to come up with alternatives to self-serving ideas that they have used in the past. Typical examples of self-talk techniques used are:

1 I am in control of my behaviour.
2 It is my responsibility to avoid putting myself in risky situations.
3 Just because a child smiles at me doesn't mean they want me to assault them.

4 If I go for a walk now the schools will be closing. I should leave it until later.

5 Maybe it's best to get out of this situation. I will go.

After getting group members to list a number of 'positive self-talk statements', from the examples earlier generated by the group, the facilitator completes the exercise by asking group members to rank the self-talk statements in their order of usefulness to each individual in the group. Advocate the notion that group members have a number of different self-talk statements.

Exercise IX

Content aim

To outline the use of covert sensitisation (CS) as an effective way to control sexual arousal.

Content objectives

1 To get group members to understand the link between sexual fantasy, masturbation and behaviour.
2 To distribute CS handouts.
3 To encourage the redirection of sexual arousal towards appropriate behaviours.

Process aim

To emphasise and develop feelings of control over sexual arousal in critical situations.

Process objectives

See 'content objectives' above.

Exercise brief

Covert sensitisation (CS) is introduced in this exercise. Group members are encouraged to employ CS techniques to counter the physical arousal experienced in response to fantasies.

The facilitator should outline to group members the link between fantasy and behaviour. Next, the idea of covert sensitisation is explained to group members. This is the pairing of any favoured fantasy with particularly unpleasant thoughts or ideas. So group members will need to think of ideas and images which they find very unpleasant. These need to be generated separately for each group member, possibly as a homework assignment. Whenever they experience fantasies or thoughts related to offending, they should try to think of the unpleasant ideas or images. Distribute handouts to interested parties and also (if available) suggest cassette tapes too. Emphasise that for covert sensitisation to be effective it is essential that the techniques are practised regularly whenever the individual experiences inappropriate fantasies. This is critical if the technique is to have an effect before or in 'high-risk' situations.

Exercise XI

Content aim

To outline the use of relapse prevention (RP) as an effective way to control sexual behaviour.

Content objectives

1 To explain the RP model to group members.
2 To get group members to generate relapse prevention strategies.
3 To get group members to identify sources of support in preventing relapses.

Process aim

To emphasise and develop feelings of control over sexual behaviour in critical situations.

Process objectives

See 'content objectives' above.

Exercise brief

In this exercise the facilitators take some of the examples of 'high-risk situations' generated in earlier exercises. Group members are then asked to:

1 List as many solutions as they can think of.
2 List the short-term and long-term consequences of each solution.
3 List the most adaptive credible responses that they would feel able to use.
4 List a number of people or agencies that could (a) monitor their behaviour; and (b) be approached for help or guidance in a crisis.

Relapse prevention is often portrayed as an approach which is separate from other cognitive behavioural approaches. Given the efficacy of relapse prevention in addressing a wide range of 'addictive behaviours' we would question this interpretation. Certainly in the context of sex offending we would argue that relapse prevention is likely to be an integral part of any effective cognitive–behavioural intervention.

Relapse prevention with sex offenders will to a large extent depend on the quality of information from the initial assessment and from the groupwork. The methods planned will need to be completed for each group member.

On completion of an intervention with sex offenders, it is also important to explain some key points to group members. First, it needs to be made clear that they are in no sense 'cured'. This point needs to be reinforced as individuals become more confident that they will not reoffend. What facilitators need to make clear is the group members will need to go on monitoring their thoughts, feeling and behaviours, that they will need to think through how to avoid or cope with 'high-risk' situations and that they will need to seek assistance when they feel their ability to avoid offending is breaking down.

INTERPERSONAL SKILLS

A proportion of sex offenders will show deficits in their social or interpersonal skills. Where this is clearly the case then practitioners may need to address these deficits. However, such skills need to be taught only when offenders have achieved a level of victim empathy and a good degree of behavioural control. In the absence of this such interventions may simply give sex offenders skills which enable them to offend more easily. For this reason we would suggest that interventions in such areas should occur after interventions to address offending.

Critically it appears that the efficacy of interventions to address such skills deficits depend on offenders being able to integrate these skills into appropriate mental frameworks (McFall, 1990; Needs, 1989). In the case of sex offenders any intervention concerned with social or interpersonal skills would need to link into overall beliefs that any sexual behaviour should be between consenting adults. Without this, such interventions are potentially damaging.

WEAKNESSES OF SELF-MANAGEMENT

Treatment programmes which have used relapse prevention methods (for example, the HM Prison Service Treatment Programme) need to lay stress on the importance of acknowledging and constructively working through any lapses (e.g. the reoccurrence of sexual fantasies about children) in self-management. In the UK this would normally involve discussing such lapses with a supervising probation officer, although it might involve other professional groups such as psychiatric nurses, social workers or, in some cases, the police.

Reliance on the offender to be motivated on their own is unlikely to be effective in a number of cases. There are a variety of possible reasons for this. First, offenders, despite frequent repetition about the need for constant vigilance can become overconfident about their ability to self-manage their behaviour.

For these reasons relapse prevention is probably most effective where it can be supplemented by external supervision, in addition to self-management techniques (Pithers, 1990).

Another factor may simply be forgetting the knowledge and techniques covered during treatment. Offenders may also be reticent about disclosing lapses to professionals because of concerns about the consequences of such disclosures. Offenders on life licences or released under some sections of the Mental Health Act are vulnerable to being detained longer or being recalled to prison or hospital. With the advent of the Criminal Justice Act (1991) this will also be true for an increasing number of released sex offenders under supervision. Even where there is no prospect of recall to prison, offenders may be concerned that disclosing lapses will lead to their children being taken into care and so on. Finally, some offenders may simply fail to disclose lapses because they are not genuinely motivated to avoid relapsing into sexual offending.

Many of the behaviours which might be of concern to a supervising officer with other offenders may be absent with sex offenders. Thus, a sex offender may be in full-time employment, a long-term relationship and be free from any substance abuse problems. In such cases looking for general patterns of unstable behaviour are unlikely to be fruitful. A more detailed account of an offender's pattern of offending is likely to be more useful.

Another fundamental aspect of external supervision is the establishment of a good network of contacts (e.g. spouse or partner, relatives, friends, social workers, community mental health teams) who are informed about the offender's pattern of relapsing. Wherever possible a network of individuals should be encouraged to both support the offender, and report any lapses to the supervising officer. How effective this approach will be depends on several factors. Some offenders may have few such contacts who are either able or willing to provide such support. In other cases it may be difficult for contacts to report lapses. Spouses might be afraid of being physically or sexually abused and therefore may not be a reliable means of monitoring lapses. Alternatively, family members may be reluctant to 'grass' on other family members where the evidence is equivocal, especially in view of the possible consequences for the offender.

SUMMARY

In this chapter we consider the treatment of sex offenders. This begins with an initial consideration of the choice between group-based and individual intervention. We then go on to consider the context of such work, both historically and politically. This is followed by a review of the practical problems involved in implementing such work, and suggested ideas and approaches to resolving or ameliorating these.

We then outline a series of group-based exercises which can be used in the treatment of sex offenders. These are divided into three main sections: (1) understanding sex offending; (2) individual offending; and (3) preventing offending. The content and process aims for each of the exercises are described. This section concludes with an exercise on relapse prevention, after which we outline some important considerations in using this approach. We discuss possible further areas of intervention which may be required, and the practical considerations involved in these. Finally, we outline some of the considerations involved in using self-management methods with sex offenders.

Bibliography

Abel, G. G. and Rouleau, J.-L. (1990). 'The nature and extent of sexual assault.' In Marshall, W. L., Laws, D. R. and Barbaree, H. E. (eds) *Handbook of Sexual Assault: Issues, Theories, and Treatment of the Offender*. New York: Plenum Press.

Abel, G. G., Barlow, D. H., Blanchard, E. B. and Guild, D. (1977). 'The components of rapist's sexual arousal.' *Archives of General Psychiatry*, 34, 895–903.

Abel, G. G., Blanchard, E. B. and Becker, J. V. (1978a). 'An integrated treatment program for rapists.' In Rada, R. (ed) *Clinical Aspects of the Rapist*. New York: Grune & Stratton.

Abel, G. G., Blanchard, E. B., Becker, J. V. and Djenderdjian, A. (1978b). 'Differentiating sexual aggressives with penile measures.' *Criminal Justice and Behaviour*, 5, 315–32.

Abel, G. G., Becker, J. V., Blanchard, E. B. and Flanangan, B. (1981). 'The behavioral assessment of rapists.' In Hays, J., Roberts, T. and Solway, K. (eds) *Violence and the Violent Individual*. Holliswood, NY: Spectrum Publications.

Abel, G. G., Becker, J. V., Cunningham-Rathner, J., Mittelman, M. S. and Rouleau, J.-L. (1988). 'Multiple paraphilic diagnoses among sex offenders.' *Bulletin of the American Academy of Psychiatry and Law*, 16, 153–68.

Abramson, L. Y., Seligman, M. E. P. and Teasdale, J. D. (1978). 'Learned Helplessness in Humans: Critique and Reformulation.' *Journal of Abnormal Psychology*, 87, 49–74.

Ajzen, I. and Fishbein, M. (1977). 'Attitude–behavior relations: A theoretical analysis and a review of empirical research.' *Psychological Bulletin*, 84, 888–918.

American Psychiatric Association (1994). *Diagnostic and Statistical Manual*, 4th edn (revised). Washington, DC: American Psychiatric Association.

Amir, M. (1971). *Patterns of Forcible Rape*. Chicago: University of Chicago Press.

Anderberg, J. (1989). 'Suicide.' In Hanson, B. and Hermern, H. (eds) *Studies in Philosophy*, Lund, Sweden: Lund University Press.

Arnold, M. B. (1960). *Emotion and Personality*, Volumes 1 and 2. New York: Columbia University Press.

Aronson, E. (1972). *The Social Animal*. San Francisco, CA: Freeman.

Asch, S. E. (1951). 'Effects of group pressure upon the modification and distortion of judgement.' In Guetzkow, H. (ed) *Groups, Leadership and Men.* Pittsburgh: Carnegie Press.

Asch, S. E. (1956). 'Studies of independence and conformity: a minority of one against a unanimous majority.' *Psychological Monographs*, 70, No. 9, Whole Number 416.

Averill, J. (1982), *Anger and Aggression: An Essay on Emotion.* New York: Springer Verlag.

Ayllon, T. and Azrin, N. (1968). *The Token Economy.* New York: Appleton Century Crofts.

Bailey, J. E. (1995). 'Lifer recalls.' Paper presented at the British Criminology Conference, Nottingham.

Baker, A. and Duncan, S. (1985). 'Child sexual abuse: a study of prevalence in Great Britain.' *Child Abuse and Neglect*, 9, 457–67.

Baker, D. (1985). 'Father–daughter incest: A study of the father.' Unpublished doctoral dissertation, University of California, San Diego.

Baker, D. and Donelly, P. G. (1986). 'Neighbourhood criminals and outsiders in two communities: indications that criminal localism varies.' *Social Science Research*, 71 (1), October.

Bandura, A. (1977). 'Self efficacy: towards a unifying theory of behavioral change.' *Psychological Review*, 84, 191–215.

Barbaree, H. E. (1990). 'Stimulus control of sexual arousal: its role in sexual assault.' In Marshall, W. L., Laws, D. R. and Barbaree, H. E. (eds) *Handbook of Sexual Assault: Issues, Theories, and Treatment of the Offender.* New York: Plenum Press.

Barbaree, H. E. and Marshall, W. L. (1989). 'Erectile responses among heterosexual child-molesters, father–daughter incest offenders and matched non-offenders: Five distinct age preference profiles.' *Canadian Journal of Behavioural Science*, 21, 70–82.

Barbaree, H. E., Marshall, W. L. and Lanthier, R. D. (1979). 'Deviant sexual arousal in rapists.' *Behaviour Research and Therapy*, 17, 215–22.

Barbaree, H. E., Marshall, W. L., Yates, E. P. and Lightfoot, L. O. (1983). 'Alcohol intoxication and deviant arousal in male social drinkers.' *Behaviour Research and Therapy*, 21, 365–73.

Barbaree, H. E., Marshall, W. L. and Connor, J. (1988). 'The social problem-solving of child molesters.' Unpublished manuscript, Queen's University, Kingston, Ontario, Canada.

Bardwick, J. M. (1979). *In Transition.* New York: Holt, Reinhart & Winston.

Bartlett, F. C. (1932). *Remembering.* Cambridge, UK: Cambridge University Press.

Baumrind, D. (1972). 'Socialization and instrumental competence in young children.' In Hartup, W. W. (ed). *The Young Child: Reviews of Research*, Vol. 2. Washington DC: National Association for the Education of Young Children.

Baxter, D. J., Marshall, W. L., Barbaree, H. E., Davidson, P. R. and Malcolm, P. B. (1984). 'Deviant sexual behavior: differentiating sex offenders by criminal and personal history, psychometric measures and sexual response.' *Criminal Justice and Behavior*, 11, 477–501.

Baxter, D. J., Barbaree, H. E. and Marshall, W. L. (1986). 'Sexual responses to consenting and forced sex in a large sample of rapists and non-rapists.' *Behaviour Research and Therapy*, 24, 513–20.

Beck, A. T. (1967). *Depression: Clinical, Experimental and Theoretical Aspects*. New York: Harper & Row.

Beck, A. T. (1991). *Cognitive Therapy and the Emotional Disorders*. London, England: Penguin Books.

Beck, A. T., Weissman, A. Lester, D. S. and Trater, L. (1974). 'The measurement of pessimism: the hopelessness scale.' *Journal of Consulting and Clinical Psychology*, 42, 861–65.

Beck, A. T., Kovacs, M and Weissman, A. S. (1975). 'Hopelessness and suicidal behavior.' *Journal of the American Medical Association*, 234, (11), 1146–9.

Beck, A. T., Kovacs, M and Weissman, A. S. (1979). 'Assessment of suicidal intention: the scale for suicide ideation.' *Journal of Consulting and Clinical Psychology*, 47, 343–50.

Beckett, R. C. (1994). 'Cognitive–behavioural treatment of sex offenders.' In Morrison, T., Erooga, M. and Beckett, R. C. (eds) *Sexual Offending against Children: Assessment and Treatment of Male Abusers*. London: Routledge.

Bee, H. L. (1995) *The Growing Child*. New York: Harper Collins.

Bellinger, D., Sloman, J., Leviton, A., Rabinowitz, M., Needleman, H. L. and Waternaux, C. (1991). 'Low level lead exposure and children's cognitive function in the preschool years.' *Pediatrics*, 87, 219–27.

Bem, D. J. (1967). 'Self perception: an alternative interpretation of cognitive dissonance phenomena.' *Psychological Review*, 74, 183–200.

Bem, D. and Funder, D. (1978). 'Predicting more of the people more of the time: assessing the personality of situations.' *Psychological Review*, 85, 485–501.

Bennett, S. R. (1985). 'Cognitive style of incestuous fathers.' Unpublished doctoral dissertation, Texas Technical University, Texas.

Berkowitz, A. R. (1983). 'Incest as related to feelings of inadequacy, impaired empathy, and early childhood memories.' Unpublished doctoral dissertation, University of Southern California, Los Angeles.

Berkowitz, L. (1962). *Aggression: A Social Psychological Analysis*. New York: McGraw Hill.

Bottomley, K. and Pease, K. (1986). *Crime and Punishment: Interpreting the Data*. Milton Keynes, UK: Open University Press.

Bowlby, J. (1969). *Attachment and Loss (Volume 1): Attachment*. New York: Basic Books.

Bowlby, J. (1988). *A Secure Base*. New York: Basic Books.

Brandon, C. (1985). 'Sex role identification in incest: an empirical analysis of the feminist theories.' Unpublished doctoral dissertation, University of Southern California, Los Angeles.

Brantigham, P. J. and Brantigham, P. L.(eds) (1981). *Environmental Criminology*. London: Sage.

Brittain, R. P. (1970) 'The Sadistic Murderer.' *Medicine Science and the Law*, 10, 198–207.

Brody, S. and Tarling, R. (1980). *Taking Offenders Out of Circulation*. London: HMSO.

Brown, A. (1989) *Groupwork* (2nd edn). London: Gower Publishing.

Burgess, A. W., Hartman, C. R., Ressler, R. K., Douglas, J. E. and McCormack,

A. (1986). 'Sexual homicide: a motivational model.' *Journal of Interpersonal Violence*, 1, 251–72.

Buss, A. H. (1961). *The Psychology of Aggression*. New York: Wiley.

Butler, S. (1978). *Conspiracy of Silence: The Trauma of Incest*. San Francisco: New Glide.

Cannon, W. B. (1915). *Bodily Changes in Pain, Hunger, Fear and Rage*. New York: Appleton-Century-Crofts.

Canter, D., Heritage, R., Davies, A., Holden, R., Kirby, S., Hancock, C., John, E., King-Johannessen, K. and McGinley, J. (1990). *Developments in Offender Profiling* (final report to the Home Office). Contract Number SC88/22/247/1. Guildford: University of Surrey.

Caspi, A., Lynam, D., Moffitt, T. E. and Silva, P. A. (1993). 'Unravelling girls' delinquency: biological, dispositional and contextual contributions to adolescent misbehavior.' *Developmental Psychology*, 29, 19–30.

Chandler, M. and Moran, T. (1990). 'Psychopathology and moral development: a comparative study of delinquent and non-delinquent youth.' *Development and Psychopathology*, 2, 227–46.

Chess, S. and Thomas, A. (1984). *Origins and Evolution of Behavior Disorders: Infancy to Early Adult Life*. New York: Brunner/Mazel.

Christiansen, K. O. (1977). 'A review of studies of criminality among twins.' In Mednick, S. A. and Christiansen, K. O. (eds) *Biosocial Bases of Criminal Behavior*. New York: Gardiner Press.

Clark, D. C. and Fawcett, J. (1992). 'Review of empirical risk factors for evaluation of the suicidal patient.' In Bongar, B. (1992) (ed.) *Suicide, Guidelines for Assessment, Management and Treatment*. Oxford: Oxford University Press.

Clark, N. K. (1993). 'Sexual offenders: an overview.' In Clark, N. K. and Stephenson, G. M. (eds) *Sexual Offenders: Context, Assessment and Treatment*. DCLP Occasional Paper No. 19. Leicester, UK: DCLP/British Psychological Society.

Collin, M. F., Halsey, C. L. and Anderson, C. L. (1991). 'Emerging developmental sequelae in the "normal" extremely low birth weight infant.' *Pediatrics*, 88, 115–20.

Conklin, J. E. (1972). *Robbery and the Criminal Justice System*. New York: J. B. Lippincott.

Cooper, D. F. and Chapman, B. (1987). *Risk Analysis for Large Projects: Models, Methods and Cases*. Chichester: Wiley.

Copson, G. (1996) 'At last some facts about offender profiling in Britain'. *Forensic Update*, 46, 3–9.

Cormier, B., Kennedy, M. and Sangowicz, J. (1962). 'Psychodynamics of father–daughter incest.' *Canadian Psychiatric Association Journal*, 7, 207–17.

Council for Science and Society (1977). *The Acceptability of Risks*. Chichester: Barry Rose Publishers.

Crighton, D. A. (1989). 'An attempt to produce an empirically based taxonomy of homicide offenders.' *Proceedings of the Prison Service Psychology Conference, Harrogate, UK*. London: Home Office Prison Service.

Crighton, D. A. (1995). 'Groupwork with sex offenders.' In Towl, G. J. (ed.) *Groupwork in Prisons*. Leicester, UK: DCLP/British Psychological Society.

Crighton, D. A. and Towl, G. J. (1995). 'Evaluation issues in groupwork.' In

Towl, G. J. (ed.) *Groupwork in Prisons*. Leicester, UK: DCLP/British Psychological Society.

Cummings, C., Gordon, J. and Marlatt, G. A. (1980). 'Strategies of prevention and prediction.' In Miller, W. R. (ed.) *The Addictive Behaviors: Treatment of Alcoholism, Drug Abuse, Smoking and Obesity*. New York: Pergamon.

Cundy, S. L. (1995). 'An evaluation of anger management work with women prisoners.' Unpublished report for HM Prison Service. Cambridge: Institute of Criminology.

Darke, J. L. (1986). 'The role of aggression and consent in the deviant sexual arousal of university males.' Unpublished doctoral dissertation, Queen's University, Kingston, Ontario.

Darke, J. L. (1990). 'Sexual aggression: achieving power through humiliation.' In Marshall, W. L., Laws, D. R. and Barbaree, H. E. (eds) *Handbook of Sexual Assault: Issues, Theories, and Treatment of the Offender*. New York: Plenum Press.

Dexter, P. (1993). 'An investigation into suicidal behaviours at HM Prison Highpoint.' Unpublished MSc thesis, University of London.

Dexter, P. and Towl, G. J. (1995). 'An investigation into suicidal behaviours in prison.' In Clark, N. K. and Stephenson, G. M. (eds) *Criminal Behaviour: Perceptions, Attributions and Rationality*. Leicester, UK: DCLP/British Psychological Society.

Diekstra, R. F. W. and Hawton, K. (eds) (1987). *Suicide in Adolescence*. Dordrecht: Martinus Nijhoff Publishers.

Dobash, R. E. and Dobash, R. (1980). *Violence against Wives: a Case against the Patriarchy*. Somerset: Open Books Publishing.

Dobash, R. E. and Dobash, R. P. (1992). *Women, Violence and Social Change*. New York: Routledge.

Dobash, R. E., Dobash, R. P. and Noaks, L.(eds) (1995). *Gender and Crime*. Cardiff: University of Wales Press.

Dollard, J. and Miller, N. E. (1950). *Personality and Psychotherapy: An Analysis in Terms of Learning, Thinking and Culture*. New York: McGraw Hill.

Dornbusch, S. M., Carlsmith, J. M., Bushwell, S. J., *et al.* (1985). 'Single parents, extended households, and the control of adolescents.' *Child Development*, 56, 326–41.

Douglas, M. (1992). *Risk and Blame: Essays in Cultural Theory*. London: Routledge.

Douglas, J. E., Ressler, R. K., Burgess, A. W. and Hartman, C. R. (1986). 'Criminal profiling from crime scene analysis.' *Behavioral Sciences and the Law*, 4, 401–21.

Dryfoos, J. (1990). *Adolescents at Risk: Prevalence and Prevention*. New York: Oxford University Press.

D'Zurilla, T. J. and Goldfried, M. R. (1971). 'Problem solving and behavior modification.' *Journal of Abnormal Psychology*, 78, 107–26.

Earls, C. M. and Marshall, W. L. (1983). 'The current state of technology in the laboratory assessment of sexual arousal patterns.' In Geer, J. G. and Stuart, I. R. (eds) *Sexual Aggression: Current Perspectives on Treatment*. New York: Van Nostrand Reinhold.

Edwards, S. S.M. (1986). 'The real risks of violence behind closed doors.' *New Law Journal*, 136, 1191–93.

Ellis, A. (1962). *Reason and Emotion in Psychotherapy*. New York: Lyle Stuart.

Ellis, A. (1976). 'Rational emotive therapy.' In Binder, V., Binder, A. and Rimland, B. (eds) *Modern Therapies*. Engelwood Cliffs, NJ: Prentice Hall.

Eron, L. D., Huesmann, L. R. and Zelli, A. (1991). 'The role of parental variables in the learning of aggression.' In Pepler, D. J. and Rubin, H. K. (eds) *The Development and Treatment of Childhood Aggression*. Hillsdale, NJ: Erlbaum.

European Collaborative Study (1991). 'Children born to women with HIV-1 infection: natural history and risk of transmission.' *The Lancet*, 337, 253–60.

Eyman, J. R. and Eyman, S. K. (1992). 'Psychological testing for potentially suicidal individuals.' In Bongar, B. (ed.) *Suicide, Guidelines for Assessment, Management and Treatment*. Oxford: Oxford University Press.

Eysenck, H. J. (1952). 'The effects of psychotherapy: an evaluation.' *Journal of Consulting Psychology*, 16, 319–24.

Farrington, D. P. (1978). 'The family backgrounds of aggressive youths.' In Hersov, L., Berger, M. and Shaffer, D. (eds) *Aggression and Anti-social Behaviour in Childhood and Adolescence*. Oxford: Pergamon.

Farrington, D. P. (1991). 'Childhood aggression and adult violence: early precursors and later life outcomes.' In Pepler, D. J. and Rubin, H. K. (eds) *The Development and Treatment of Childhood Aggression*. Hillsdale, NJ: Erlbaum.

Farrington, D. P. (1993). 'The challenge of teenage anti-social behaviour.' Paper prepared for the Martach Castle Conference on ' Youth in the Year 2000'.

Farrington, D. P. and West, D. J. (1990). 'The Cambridge study in delinquent development: a long term follow up of 411 London males.' In Kaiser, G. and Kerner, H. J. (eds) *Criminality: Personality, Behaviour, Life History*. Heidelberg: Springer Verlag.

Fenton, G. W., Fenwick, P. B.C., Fergusson, W. and Lamb, C. T. (1978). 'The contingent negative variation in antisocial behaviour: a pilot study of Broadmoor patients.' *British Journal of Psychiatry*, 132, 368–77.

Fergusson, D. M., Horwood, L. J. and Lynskey, M. T. (1993). 'Maternal smoking before and after pregnancy: effects on behavioural outcomes in middle childhood.' *Pediatrics*, 92, 815–22.

Feshbach, S. (1970). 'Aggression.' In Mussen, P. H. (ed.) *Carmichael's Manual of Child Psychology*, Volume 2, 3rd edn. New York: Wiley.

Festinger, L. (1957). *A Theory of Cognitive Dissonance*. Evanston, IL: Row Peterson.

Finkelhor, D. (1979). *Sexually Victimized Children*. New York: Free Press.

Finkelhor, D. (1984). *Child Sexual Abuse: New Theory and Research*. New York: Free Press.

Finkelhor, D. (1986). *A Sourcebook on Child Sexual Abuse*. Newbury Park, CA: Sage.

Fishbein, M. (1967). 'Attitude and the prediction of behavior.' In Fishbein, M. (ed.) *Readings in Attitude Theory and Measurement*. New York: Wiley.

Floyd, R. L., Rimer, B. K., Giovino, G. A., Mullen, P. D. and Sullivan, S. E. (1993). 'A review of smoking in pregnancy: effects on pregnancy outcomes and cessation efforts.' *Annual Review of Public Health*, 14, 379–411.

Fredrickson, R. M. (1981). 'Incest: Families sexual abuse and its relationship to pathology, sex role orientation, attitudes towards women, and authoritarianism.' Unpublished doctoral dissertation, University of Minnesota.

Freund, K. (1967). 'Erotic preference in pedophilia.' *Behaviour Research and Therapy*, 5, 339–48.

Freund, K. (1981). 'Assessment of pedophilia.' In Cook, M. and Howells, K. (eds) *Adult Sexual Interest in Children*. London: Academic Press.

Gabor, T. (1986). *The Prediction of Criminal Behaviour*. Toronto: University of Toronto Press.

Gabor, T., Baril, M., Cusson, M., Elie, D., LeBlanc, M. and Normandeau, A. (1987). *Armed Robbery, Cops, Robbers and Victims*. Springfield, IL: C. C.Thomas.

Ganong, W. F. (1991). *Review of Medical Physiology* (15th edn). New Haven, Connecticut: Appleton Lange.

Garbarino, J., Kostelny, K. and Dubrow, N. (1991). *No Place to be a Child: Growing Up In A War Zone*. Lexington, MA: Lexington Books.

Gebhard, P., Gagnon, J., Pomeroy, W. and Christenson, C. (1965). *Sex Offenders: An Analysis of Types*. New York: Harper & Row.

Geer, J. H. and Fuhr, R. (1976). 'Cognitive factors in sexual arousal: the role of distraction.' *Journal of Consulting and Clinical Psychology*, 44, 238–43.

Gelles, R. J. (1982). 'Domestic criminal violence.' In Wolfgang, M. E. and Weiner, N. A. (eds) *Criminal Violence*. London: Sage Publications.

Gendreau, P., Freedman, N. L., Wilde, G. J.S. and Scott, G. D. (1972). 'Changes in EEG alpha frequency and evoked response latency during solitary confinement.' *Journal of Abnormal Psychology*, 79, 54–9.

Gerard, H. B. and Greenbaum, C. (1962). 'Attitudes toward an agent of uncertainty reduction.' *Journal of Personality*, 30, 485–95.

Getz, W. L., Allen, D. B., Keith-Myers, R. and Lindler, K. C. (1987). *Brief Counselling with Suicidal Persons*. Lexington, MA: Lexington Books.

Gilbert, P. (1984). *Depression, from Psychology to Brain State*. London: Lawrence Erlbaum Associates.

Gillin, J. (1946). *The Wisconsin Prisoner*. Madison: University of Wisconsin Press.

Goldstein, A. and Foa, E. B. (1980). *Handbook of Behavioral Interventions – A Clinical Guide*. New York: Wiley.

Gottman, J. M. (1986). 'The world of coordinated play: same and cross-sex friendships in young children.' In Gottman, J. M. and Parker, J. G. (eds) *Conversations of Friends. Speculations on Affective Development*. Cambridge, UK: Cambridge University Press.

Groth, N. A. (1979). *Men who Rape: The Psychology of the Offender*. New York: Plenum.

Groth, N. A. and Burgess, A. W. (1977). 'Rape: A sexual deviation.' *American Journal of Orthopsychiatry*, 47(3), 400–6.

Gunn, J., Maden, A. and Swinton, M. (1991). 'Treatment needs of prisoners with psychiatric disorders.' *British Medical Journal*, 303, 338–41.

Hall, J. N. and Baker, R. D. (1986). 'Token economies and schizophrenia: a review.' In Kerr, A. and Snaith, R. P. (eds) *Contemporary Issues in Schizophrenia*. London: Gaskell.

Hare, R. D. (1985). 'A comparison of procedures for the assessment of psychopathy.' *Journal of Consulting and Clinical Psychology*, 53, 7–16.

Hare, R. D. (1986). 'Twenty years of experience with the Cleckley psychopath.' In Reid, W. H., Dorr, D., Walker, J. and Bonner, J. W. (eds) *Unmasking the*

Psychopath: Antisocial Personality and Related Syndromes. New York: Norton.

Harris, T. (1982). *The Red Dragon*. London: Bodley Head Ltd.

Harrison, G. (1995). 'Mental health and risk management.' Symposium presented at the Institute for the Study and Treatment of Delinquency annual conference, University of Nottingham, April.

Hawton, K. (1986). Suicide and Attempted Suicide among Children and Adolescents. Beverly Hills, CA: Sage.

Hawton, K., Salkovkis, P. M., Kirk, J. and Clark, D. M. (1989). *Cognitive Behaviour Therapy for Psychiatric Problems: A Practical Guide*. Oxford: Oxford University Press.

Heagarty, M. C. (1991). 'America's lost children: whose responsibility?' *Journal of Pediatrics*, 118, 8–10.

Heider, F. (1944). 'Social perception and phenomenal causality.' *Psychological Review*, 51, 358–74.

Heider, F. (1958). *The Psychology of Interpersonal Relations*. New York: Wiley.

Herman, J. (1981). *Father–Daughter Incest*. Cambridge, MA: Harvard University Press.

Herrington, L. H. (1982). *Final Report of the President's Task Force on Victims of Crime (Herrington, L. H. – Chairperson)*. Library of Congress report number 82-24146. Washington, DC: The White House.

Hetherington, E. M. (1989). 'Coping with family transitions: winners, losers and survivors.' *Child Development*, 60, 1–14.

Hey, J. D. (1979). *Uncertainty in Microeconomics*. Oxford: M. Robertson and Co.

HM Prison Service (1994). *Core Treatment Programme for Sex Offenders* (revised version). London: HM Prison Service.

HM Prison Service (1995a). *Anger Management Course Training Manual* (revised version). London: HM Prison Service.

HM Prison Service (1995b). *Briefing, No. 87*. London: Central Office of Information.

Hofferth, S. L. (1985). 'Updating children's life course.' *Journal of Marriage and the Family*, 47, 93–115.

Holmes, R. M. (1990). *Profiling Violent Crimes*. Newbury Park, CA: Sage.

Holmes, R. M. and DeBurger, J. (1988). *Serial Murder*. Newbury Park, CA: Sage.

Howells, K. (1979). 'Some meanings of children for paedophiles.' In Cook, M. and Wilson, F. (eds) *Love and Attraction*. Oxford, UK: Pergamon.

Hsu, L. K. G., Wisner, K., Richey, E. T. and Goldstein, C. (1985). 'Is juvenile delinquency related to an abnormal EEG? A study of abnormalities in juvenile delinquents and adolescent psychiatric inpatients.' *Journal of the American Academy of Child Psychiatry*, 24, 310–15.

Hutchings, B. and Mednick, S. A. (1975). 'Registered criminality in the adoptive and biological parents of registered male criminal adoptees.' In Fieve, R. R., Rosenthal, D. and Brill, H. (eds) *Genetic Research in Psychiatry*. Baltimore: Johns Hopkins University Press.

Hutto, C., Parks, W. P. and Lai, S. (1991). 'A hospital based prospective study of perinatal infection with human immunodeficiency virus type 1.' *Journal of Pediatrics*, 118, 347–53.

Inch, H., Rowland, P. and Seliman, A. (1995). 'Deliberate self-mutilation in a young offender institution.' *Journal of Forensic Psychiatry*, 6(1), 161–71.

James, W. (1890). *The Principles of Psychology*. Cambridge, MA: Harvard University Press.

Jarvick, L. F., Klodin, V. and Matsuyama, S. S. (1973). 'Human aggression and the extra Y chromosome: fact or fantasy.' *American Psychologist*, 28, 674–82.

Jones, E. E. and Harris, V. A. (1967). 'The attribution of attitudes.' *Journal of Experimental Social Psychology*, 3, 1–24.

Jones, E. E. and Nisbett, R. E. (1971). 'The actor and observer: divergent perceptions of the causes of behavior.' In Jones, E. E., Kanouse, D. E., Kelley, H. H., Nisbett, R. E., Valins, S. and Weiner, B. (eds) *Attribution: Perceiving the Causes of Behavior*. Morristown, NJ: General Learning Press.

Jones, M. C. (1924). 'The elimination of children's fears.' *Journal of Experimental Psychology*, 7, 382–90.

Kahneman, D. and Tversky, A. (1973). 'On the psychology of prediction.' *Psychological Review*, 80, 237–51.

Kahneman, D., Slovic, P. and Tversky, A. (eds) (1982). *Judgment under Uncertainty: Heuristical Biases*. Cambridge: Cambridge University Press.

Kaplan, M. S. (1985). 'The impact of parolees' perceptions of confidentiality on the reporting of their urges to interact sexually with children.' Unpublished doctoral disertation. New York University.

Kelley, H. H. (1967). 'Attribution theory in social psychology.' In Levine, D. (ed.), *Nebraska Symposium on Motivation*. 15, 192–238.

Kelley, H. H. (1971). 'Causal schemata and the attribution process.' In Jones, E. E., Kanouse, D. E., Kelley, H. H., Nisbett, R. E., Valins, S. and Weiner, B. (eds) *Attribution: Perceiving the Causes of Behavior*. Morristown, NJ: General Learning Press.

Kelly, G. A. (1955). *The Psychology of Personal Constructs*. New York: Norton.

Kelly, G. A. (1961). 'Suicide: the personal construct point of view.' In Farterow, N. and Shneidman, E. (eds) *The Cry for Help*. New York: McGraw Hill.

Kelly, L. (1991). *Surviving Sexual Violence*. Cambridge, UK: Polity Press.

Kiesler, C. A., Nisbett, R. E. and Zanna, M. P. (1969). 'On inferring one's beliefs from one's behavior.' *Journal of Personality and Social Psychology*, 11, 321–27.

Kirkland, K. and Bauer, C. (1982). 'MMPI traits of incestuous fathers.' *Journal of Criminal Psychology*, 38, 645–9.

Knight, R. A. and Prentky, R. A. (1990). 'Classifying sexual offenders: the development and corroboration of taxonomic models.' In Marshall, W. L., Laws, D. R. and Barbaree, H. E. (eds) *Handbook of Sexual Assault: Issues, Theories, and Treatment of the Offender*. New York: Plenum Press.

Kohlberg, L. (1964). 'Development of moral character and ideology.' In Hoffman, M. L. and Hoffman, L. W. (eds) *Review of Child Development Research* (Volume 1). New York: Russell Sage Foundation.

Kohlberg, L. (1966). 'A cognitive–developmental analysis of chilren's sex-role concepts and attitudes.' In Maccoby, E. E. (ed.) *The Development of Sex Differences*. Stanford, CA, Stanford University Press.

Kohlberg, L. (1981). *Essays on Moral Development, Volume 1. The Philosophy of Moral Development*. New York: Harper and Row.

Kopp, C. B. (1983). 'Risk factors in development.' In Haith, M. M. and Campos,

J. J. (eds) *Handbook of Child Psychology: Infancy and Developmental Psychobiology* (Volume 2). New York: Wiley.

Koss, M. P., Leonard, K. E., Beezley, D. A. and Oros, C. J. (1985). 'Nonstranger sexual aggression: A psychological study of the characteristics of undetected offenders.' *Sex Roles*, 12(9/10), 981–91.

Lange, J. S. (1931). *Crime as Destiny*. London: Allen & Unwin.

Langevin, R., Handy, L., Day, D. and Russon, A. (1985). 'Are incestuous fathers pedophilic, aggressive and alcoholic?' In Langevin, R. (ed.) *Erotic Preference, Gender Identity and Aggression*. Hillsdale, NJ: Erlbaum.

LaPierre, R. T. (1934). 'Attitudes vs actions.' *Social Forces*, 13, 230–7.

Lazarus, R. S. (1966). *Psychological Stress and the Coping Process*. New York: McGraw Hill.

Leaper, C. (1991). 'Influence and involvement in children's discourse: age, gender, and partner effects.' *Child Development*, 62, 797–811.

Lee, R. N. (1982). 'Analysis of the characteristics of incestuous fathers.' Unpublished doctoral dissertation, University of Texas at Austin.

Lester, D. (1979). 'The violent offender,' In Toch, H. (ed.) *Psychology of Crime and Criminal Justice*. New York: Holt, Rinehart & Winston.

Levenson, H. (1976). 'Locus of control: a multidimensional view.' In Lefcourt, H. M. (ed.) *Locus of Control, Current Trends in Theory and Research*. New York: Wiley.

Liebling, A. (1992). *Suicides in Prison*. London: Routledge.

Lingham, R. (1995). 'Mental health and risk management.' Symposium presented at the Institute for the Study and Treatment of Delinquency annual conference, University of Nottingham, April.

Loeber, R. and Dishion, T. (1983). 'Early predictors of male delinquency: a review.' *Psychological Bulletin*, 94, 68–99.

Luhmann, N. (1993). *Risk: a Sociological Theory*. Translation by Rhodes Barrett. New York: A. de Gruyter.

Lustig, N., Dresser, J., Spellman, S. and Murray, T. (1966). 'Incest: A family group survival pattern.' *Archives of General Psychiatry*, 14, 31–9.

McCarthy, J. and Hardy, J. (1993). 'Age at first birth and birth outcomes.' *Journal of Research on Adolescence*, 3, 374–92.

McClintock, F. H. and Gibson, E. (1961), *Robbery in London*, London: Macmillan.

McClurg, G. (1996). 'A descriptive study of child sexual abusers.' *Forensic Update*, 44, 18–22. Leicester, UK: British Psychological Society.

Maccoby, E. E. (1980). *Social Development. Psychological Growth and Parent–Child Relationships*. New York: Harcourt Brace Jovanovich.

Maccoby, E. E. and Jacklin, C. N. (1987). 'Gender segregation in childhood.' In Reese, H. W. (ed.) *Advances in Child Development and Behavior* (Volume 20). Orlando FL: Academic Press.

Maccoby, E. E. and Martin, J. A. (1983). 'Socialisation in the context of the family: parent–child interaction.' In Hetherington, E. M. (ed.) *Handbook of Child Psychology: Socialisation, Personality and Development* (Volume 4). New York: Wiley.

McCord, J. (1982). 'A longitudinal view of the relationship between parental absence and crime.' In Gunn, J. and Farrington, D. P. (eds) *Abnormal Offenders, Delinquency and the Criminal Justice System*. London: Wiley.

McCord, J. (1986). 'Instigation and insulation: how families affect anti-social aggression.' In Olweus, D., Block, J. and Radke-Yarrow, M. (eds) *Development of Antisocial and Prosocial Behavior: Research, Theories, and Issues*. New York: Academic Press.

MacCulloch, M. J., Snowden, P. R., Wood, P. J. W. and Mills, H. E. (1983). 'Sadistic fantasy, sadistic behaviours and offending.' *British Journal of Psychiatry*, 143, 20–9.

McFall, R. M. (1990) 'The enhancement of social skills: an information-processing analysis.' In Marshall, W. L., Laws, D. R. and Barbaree, H. E. (eds) *Handbook of Sexual Assault: Issues, Theories and Treatment of the Offender*. New York: Plenum.

McGrath, R. (1990). 'Assessment of sexual aggressors: practical clinical interviewing strategies.' *Journal of Interpersonal Violence*, 5, 507–19.

Maisch, H. (1972). *Incest*. New York: Stein & Day.

Malamuth, N. M. and Check, J. V. P. (1980). 'Penile tumescence and perceptual responses to rape as a function of victims' perceived reactions.' *Journal of Applied Social Psychology*, 10, 528–47.

Malamuth, N. M. and Check, J. V. P. (1983). 'Sexual arousal to rape depictions: individual differences.' *Journal of Abnormal Psychology*, 92, 55–67.

Marshall, W. L. and Barbaree, H. E. (1990a). 'An integrated theory of the etiology of sexual offending.' In Marshall, W. L., Laws, D. R. and Barbaree, H. E. (eds) *Handbook of Sexual Assault: Issues, Theories, and Treatment of the Offender*. New York: Plenum Press.

Marshall, W. L. and Barbaree, H. E. (1990b). 'Outcome of comprehensive cognitive–behavioral treatment programs.' In Marshall, W. L., Laws, D. R. and Barbaree, H. E. (eds) *Handbook of Sexual Assault: Issues, Theories, and Treatment of the Offender*. New York: Plenum Press.

Marshall, W. L., Bates, L. and Ruhl, M. (1984). Hostility in sex offenders. Unpublished manuscript, Queen's Univeristy, Kingston, Ontario.

Marshall, W. L., Barbaree, H. E. and Christophe, D. (1986). 'Sexual preferences for age of victims and type of behaviour.' *Canadian Journal of Behavioural Science*, 18, 424–39.

Marshall, W. L., Laws, D. R. and Barbaree, H. E. (eds) (1990) *Handbook of Sexual Assault: Issues, Theories, and Treatment of the Offender*. New York: Plenum Press.

Maslow, A. (1970), *Motivation and Personality, Second Edition*. New York: Harper & Row.

Masserman, J. H. (1943). *Behavior and Neurosis: An Experimental Psychoanalytic Approach to Psychobiological Principles*. Chicago: University of Chicago Press.

Mednick, S. A., Volavka, J., Gabrielli, W. F. and Itil, T. M. (1981). 'EEG as a predictor of anti-social behavior.' *Criminology*, 19, 219–29.

Meehl, P. E. (1973). 'Why I do not attend case conferences.' In Meehl, P. E. (ed.) *Psycho-diagnosis. Selected Papers*. Minneapolis: University of Minnesota Press.

Megargee, E. (1966). 'Undercontrolled and overcontrolled personality types in extreme antisocial aggression.' *Psychological Monographs*, 80, Number (611).

Megargee, E. (1976). 'The prediction of dangerous behavior.' *Criminal Justice and Behavior*, 3, 3–21.

Meichenbaum, D. (1972). 'Clinical implications of modifying what clients say to themselves.' *Research Reports in Psychology*, no. 42. Waterloo, Ontario: University of Waterloo.

Meichenbaum, D. (1975). 'Self-instructional methods.' In Kanfer, F. H. and Goldstein, A. P. (eds) *Helping People Change: a Textbook of Methods*. New York: Pergamon.

Meichenbaum, D. (1977). *Cognitive–behavior Modification*. New York: Plenum Press.

Milgram, S. (1963). 'Behavioral study of obedience.' *Journal of Abnormal and Social Psychology*, 67, 371–8.

Miron, M. S. and Douglas, J. E. (1979). 'Threat analysis: the psycholinguistic approach.' *FBI Law Enforcement Bulletin*, 49, 5–9.

Mischel, W. (1968). *Personality and Assessment*. New York: Wiley.

Mischel, W. (1970). 'Sex typing and socialization.' In Mussen, P. H. (ed.). *Carmichael's Manual of Child Psychology*, (Volume 2). New York: Wiley.

Monahan, J. (1981). 'The clinical prediction of violent behavior.' *Crime and Delinquency Issues: A Monograph Series*. Washington, DC: Department of Health and Human Sciences.

Monahan, J. and Steadman, H. J. (1994). *Violence and Mental Disorder: Developments in Risk Assessment*. Chicago: University of Chicago Press.

Monroe, R. (1978). *Brain Dysfunction in Aggressive Criminals*. Lexington, MA: Heath Books.

Morgan, H. G. and Owen, J. H. (1990). *Persons at Risk of Suicide. Guidelines on Good Clinical Practice*. Nottingham: Boots PLC.

Morris, T. and Blom-Cooper, L. (1967). 'Homicide in England.' In Wolfgang, M. E. (ed.) *Studies in Homicide*. New York: Harper & Row.

Moser, K. A., Fox, A. J. and Jones, D. R. (1984). 'Unemployment and mortality in the OPCS longitudinal study.' *Lancet*, ii, 1324–8.

Moser, K. A., Goldblatt, P., Fox, J. and Jones, D. (1990). 'Unemployment and mortality.' In Goldblatt, P. (ed.) *Longitudinal Study 1971–81: Mortality and Social Organisation*. OPCS LS Series. London: HMSO.

Mowrer, O. H. and Mowrer, W. M., (1938) 'Enuresis: a method for its study and treatment.' *American Journal of Orthopsychiatry*, 8, 436–59

Murphy, W. D. (1990). 'Assessment and modification of cognitive distortions in sex offenders.' In Marshall, W. L., Laws, D. R. and Barbaree, H. E. (eds) *Handbook of Sexual Assault: Issues, Theories, and Treatment of the Offender*. New York: Plenum Press.

Murphy, W. D. and Barbaree, H. E. (1988). *Assessments of Sexual Offenders by Measurements of Erectile Response: An Examination of their Psychometric Properties*. Washington, DC: National Institute of Mental Health.

National Center for Health Statistics (1992). 'Advance report of final mortality statistics 1989.' *NCHS Monthly Vital Statistics Report*, 40, (8) Supplement.

National Committee for the Prevention of Child Abuse (1978). *Basic Facts about Child Sexual Abuse*. Chicago: Author.

Needs, A. P. C. (1988). 'The subjective context of social difficulty.' Unpublished D Phil thesis, University of York.

Needs, A. P. C. (1989). 'The lifer assessment manual.' Unpublished Home Office Prison Service manuscript.

Needs, A. P. C. (1995). 'Social skills training.' In Towl, G. J. (ed.) *Groupwork in Prisons*. Leicester, UK: British Psychological Society.

Neisser, U. (1967). *Cognitive Psychology*. New York: Appleton Century Crofts.

Neisser, U. (1976). *Cognition and Reality*. San Francisco: W. H.Freeman.

Nichols, H. R. and Mollinder, I. (1984). *Multiphasic Sex Inventory Manual*. Tacoma, WA: Nichols & Mollinder.

Nisbett, R. and Ross, L. (1980). *Human Inference: Strategies and Shortcomings of Social Judgement*. Engelwood Cliffs, NJ: Prentice Hall.

Nisbett, R. E., Borgida, E., Crandall, R. and Reed, H. (1982). 'Popular induction: information is not necessarily informative.' In Kahneman, D., Slovic, P. and Tversky, A., (eds) *Judgment under Uncertainty: Heuristical Biases*. Cambridge: Cambridge University Press.

Novaco, R. W. (1975). *Anger Control: The Development and Evaluation of an Experimental Treatment*. Lexington, MA: DC Heath and Company.

Novaco, R. W. (1980). *Novaco Anger Scale*. Irvine, CA: Department of Psychology, University of California.

Novaco, R. W. (1986). 'Anger as a clinical and social problem.' In Blanchard, R. and Blanchard, C. (eds) *Advances in the Study of Aggression*, (Volume 2). New York: Academic Press.

Novaco, R. W. and Welsh, W. N. (1989). 'Anger disturbances: cognitive mediation and clinical prescriptions.' In Howells, K. and Hollin, C. R. *Clinical Approaches to Violence*. Chichester: Wiley.

Oatley, K. (1992). *Best Laid Schemes, the Psychology of Emotions*. Cambridge: Cambridge University Press.

Offord, D. R., Boyle, M. H. and Racine, Y. A. (1991). 'The epidemiology of antisocial behavior in childhood and adolescence.' In Pepler, D. J. and Rubin, H. K. (eds) *The Development and Treatment of Childhood Aggression*. Hillsdale, NJ: Erlbaum.

O'Leary, K. D. and Wilson, G. T. (1975). *Behavior Therapy: Application and Outcome*. Engelwood Cliffs, NJ: Prentice Hall.

Olson, V. A. (1982). 'An exploratory study of incest family interaction.' Doctoral dissertation, California School of Professional Psychology, Los Angeles. *Dissertation Abstracts International*, 43.

Olson, H. C., Sampson, P. D., Barr, H., Streissgarth, A. P. and Bookstein, F. L. (1992). 'Prenatal exposure to alcohol and school problems in late childhood: a longitudinal prospective study.' *Development and Psychopathology*, 4, 341–59.

Olson, J. C. (1996). 'Psychological profiling: does it actually work?' *Forensic Update* 46, 10–13.

Owens, G. and Ashcroft, J. B. (1982). 'Functional analysis in applied psychology.' *British Journal of Clinical Psychology*, 21, 181–9.

Parker, H. (1984). 'Intrafamilial sexual child abuse: A study of the abusive father.' Unpublished doctoral dissertation, University of Utah.

Parker, H. and Parker, S. (1986). 'Father–daughter sexual abuse: An emerging perspective.' *American Journal of Orthopsychiatry*, 56, 531–49.

Patterson, G. R. (1980). 'Mothers: The unacknowledged victims.' *Monographs of the Society for Research in Child Development*, 45, (Serial Number 186).

Pavlov, I. P. (1927). *Conditioned Reflexes*. (G. V.Anrep, Translation). New York: Oxford University Press.

Petit, G. S. Bakshi, A., Dodge, K. A. *et al.* (1990). 'The emergence of social dominance in young boys' play groups: developmental differences and behavioral correlates.' *Developmental Psychology*, 26, 1017–25.

Pfeffer, C. R. (1986). *The Suicidal Child*. New York: Guilford Press.

Philips, P. (1980). 'Characteristics and typology of the journey to crime.' In Georges-Abeyie, D. E. and Harris, K. D. (eds) *Crime: a Spatial Perspective*. New York: Columbia University Press.

Piaget, J. (1932). *The Moral Judgement of the Child*. New York: Macmillan.

Pithers, W. D. (1990). 'Relapse prevention with sexual aggressors: a method for enhancing therapeutic gain and enhancing external supervision.' In Marshall, W. L., Laws, D. R. and Barbaree, H. E. (eds) *Handbook of Sexual Assault: Issues, Theories, and Treatment of the Offender*. New York: Plenum Press.

Platt, S. (1984). 'Unemployment and suicidal behavior.' *Social Science and Medicine*, 19 (2), 93–115.

Platt, S. and Kreitman, N. (1984). 'Unemployment and Parasuicide in Edinburgh 1968–1982.' *British Medical Journal*, 289, 1029–32.

Price, R. H., Glickstein, M., Horton, D. L. and Bailey, R. (1982). *Principles of Psychology*. New York: Holt Rinehart & Winston.

Quinn, T. M. (1984). 'Father–daughter incest: An ecological model.' Unpublished doctoral dissertation, University of California, Fresno, CA.

Quinsey, V. L. and Bergersen, S. G. (1976). 'Instructional control of penile circumference in assessment of sexual preference.' *Behavior Therapy*, 7, 489–93.

Quinsey, V. L. and Chaplin, T. C. (1988). 'Preventing faking in phallometric assessments of sexual preference.' In Prentky, R. and Quinsey, V. L. (eds) *Human Sexual Aggression: Current Perspectives*. New York: Annals of the New York Academy of Sciences.

Quinsey, V. L. and Earls, C. M. (1990). 'The modification of sexual preference.' In Marshall, W. L., Laws, D. R. and Barbaree, H. E. (eds) *Handbook of Sexual Assault: Issues, Theories, and Treatment of the Offender*. New York: Plenum Press.

Quinsey, V. L., Steinman, C. M., Bergersen, S. G. and Holmes, T. F. (1975). 'Penile circumference, skin conductance, and ranking responses of child molesters and "normals" to sexual and non-sexual visual stimuli.' *Behavior Therapy*, 6, 213–19.

Quinsey, V. L. and Chaplin, T. C., and Varney, G. (1981). 'A comparison of rapists' and non-sex offenders' sexual preferences for mutually consenting sex, rape and physical abuse of women.' *Behavioral Assessment*, 3, 127–35.

Rachman, S. J. and Teasdale, J. (1969). *Aversion Therapy and Behavior Disorders: An Analysis*. Coral Gables, FL: University of Miami Press.

Raine, A. (1989). 'Evoked potentials and psychopathy.' *International Journal of Psychophysiology*, 4, 277–87.

Reading, R. Raybould, S. and Jarvis, S. (1993). 'Deprivation, low birth weight, and children's height: a comparison between rural and urban areas.' *British Medical Journal*, 307, 1458–62.

Ressler, R. K., Douglas, J. E., Groth, A. N. and Burgess, A. W. (1980). 'Offender profiling: a multidisciplinary approach.' *FBI Law Enforcement Bulletin*, 49, 16–20.

Ressler, R. K., Burgess, A. W., Douglas, J. E. and Depue, R. L. (1985). 'Criminal profiling research on homicide.' In Burgess, A. W. (ed.) *Rape and Sexual Assault: a Research Handbook*. New York: Garland.

Ressler, R. K., Burgess, A. W. and Douglas, J. E. (1993). *Sexual Homicide: Patterns and Motives*. London: Simon & Schuster Ltd.

Riccuti, H. N. (1993). 'Nutrition and mental development.' *Current Directions in Psychological Science*, 2, 43–6.

Rose, S., Kamin, L. J. and Lewontin, R. C. (1984). *Not in our Genes: Biology, Ideology and Human Nature*. Harmondsworth: Penguin.

Ross, R. R., Fabiano, E. A. and Ewles, C. D. (1988). 'Reasoning and rehabilitation.' *International Journal of Offender Therapy and Comparative Criminology*, 32, 29–36.

Rowe, D. (1983). 'Biometric genetic models of self-reported delinquent behaviour: a twin study.' *Behavioral Genetics*, 13, 473–89.

Rowe, D. C. and Osgood, D. W. (1984). 'Heredity and sociological theories of delinquency: a reconsideration.' *American Sociological Review*, 49, 526–40.

Russell, D. E. H. (1975). *The Politics of Rape: The Victim's Perspective*. New York: Stein & Day.

Russell, D. E. H. (1984). *Sexual Exploitation: Rape, Child Sexual Abuse, and Workplace Harassment*. Beverly Hills, CA: Sage.

Rutter, M. (1972). 'Relationships between child and adult psychiatric disorder.' *Acta Psychiatrica Scandinavica*, 48, 3–21.

Rutter, M. (1973). 'Why are London children so disturbed?' *Proceedings of the Royal Society of Medicine*, 66, 1221–5.

Rutter, M., Birch, H. G., Thomas, A. and Chess, S. (1964). 'Temperamental characteristics in infancy and the later development of behavioural disorders.' *British Journal of Psychiatry*, 110, 651–61.

Ryan, W. (1971). *Blaming the Victim*. New York: Random House.

Salter, A. C. (1988). *Treating Child Sex Offenders and Victims: A Practical Guide*. Newbury Park, CA: Sage.

Sampson, E. E. and Insko, C. A. (1964). 'Cognitive consistency and performance in the autokinetic situation.' *Journal of Abnormal and Social Psychology*, 68, 184–92.

Saunders, B., McClure, S. and Murphy, S. (1986). *Final report: Profile of Incest Perpetrators Indicating Treatability – Part 1*. Charleston, SC: Crime Victims Research and Treatment Center.

Schacter, S. (1951). 'Deviation, rejection and communication.' *Journal of Abnormal and Social Psychology*, 46, 190–207.

Schacter, S. and Singer, J. E. (1962). 'Cognitive, social and physiological determinants of emotional states.' *Psychological Review*, 69, 379–99.

Schaefer, E. S. (1989). 'Dimensions of mother–infant interaction: measurement, stability, and predictive validity.' *Infant Behavior and Development*, 12, 379–93.

Schlesinger, L. B. and Revitch, E. (1980) 'The criminal fantasy technique: a comparison of sex offenders and substance abusers.' *Journal of Clinical Psychology*, 37, 210–18.

Schonfeld, I. S., Shaffer, D., O'Conner, P. and Portny, S. (1988). 'Conduct disorder and cognitive functioning: testing three causal hypotheses.' *Child Development*, 59, 993–1007.

Scott, R. L. and Stone, D. (1986). 'MMPI profile constellation in incest families.' *Journal of Consulting and Clinical Psychology*, 54, 364–8.

Scully, D. (1990). *Understanding Sexual Violence: A Study of Convicted Rapists*. Boston: Unwin Hyman.

Segal, Z. V. and Marshall, W. L. (1986). 'Discrepancies between self-efficacy predictions and actual performance in a population of rapists and child molesters.' *Cognitive Therapy and Research*, 10(3), 363–76.

Segal, Z. and Stermac, L. E. (1984). 'A measure of rapists' attitudes towards women.' *International Journal of Law and Psychiatry*, 7, 437–40.

Shapiro, M. B. (1961). 'A method of measuring psychological changes specific to the individual psychiatric patient.' *British Journal of Medical Psychology*, 34, 151–5.

Sherif, M. (1935). 'A study of some social factors in perception.' *Archives of Psychology*, 22, No. 187.

Shneidman, E. S. (1992). 'What do suicides have in common? Summary of the psychological approach.' In Bongar, B. (ed.) *Suicide, Guidelines for Assessment, Management and Treatment*. Oxford: Oxford University Press.

Skinner, B. F. (1971). *Beyond Freedom and Dignity*. New York: Knopf.

Slovic, D., Fischoff, B. and Lichenstein, S. (1976). In Carrol, J.S. and Payne, J. W. (eds) *Cognition and Social Behaviour*. Hillside, N.J., Erlbaum.

Simons, R. L., Robertson, J. F., and Downs, W. R. (1989). 'The nature of the association between parental rejection and delinquent behavior.' *Journal of Youth and Adolescence*, 18, 297–309.

Smith, C. A. and Lazarus, R. S. (1993). 'Appraisal components, core relational themes and emotions.' In Frijda, N. H. (ed.) *Appraisal and Beyond, the Issue of Cognitive Determinants of Emotion, Cognition and Emotion*, special issue. Hove, UK: Lawrence Erlbaum Associates.

Smith, L. L., Smith, J. N. and Beckner, B. N. (1995). 'An anger management workshop for women inmates.' *Families in Society: The Journal of Contemporary Human Services*. Utah: The University of Utah.

Snarey, J. R. (1985). 'Cross-cultural universality of social–moral development: a critical review of Kohlbergian research.' *Psychological Bulletin*, 97, 202–32.

Spielberger, C. D. (1988). *State–Trait Anger Expression Inventory*, research edition, professional manual. Miami, Florida: Psychological Assessment Resources.

Spielberger, C. D., Reheiser, E. C. and Sydeman, S. J. (1995). 'Measuring the experience, expression, and control of anger.' In Kassinove, H. (ed.). *Anger Disorders: Definition, Diagnosis and Treatment*. Washington, DC: Taylor & Francis.

Steadman, H. J. (1987). 'How well can we predict violence for adults? A review of the literature and some commentary.' In Dutile, F. N. and Foust, C. H. (eds) *The Prediction of Criminal Violence*. Springfield: C. C. Thomas.

Stearns, C. Z. and Stearns, P. N. (1986). *Anger, the Struggle for Emotional Control in America's History*. Chicago: University of Chicago Press.

Stermac, L. E. and Quinsey, V. L. (1986). 'Social competence among rapists.' *Behavioral Assessment*, 8, 171–85.

Stermac, L. E., Segal, Z. V. and Gillis, R. (1990). 'Social and cultural factors in sexual assault.' In Marshall, W. L., Laws, D. R. and Barbaree, H. E. (eds), *Handbook of Sexual Assault: Issues, Theories, and Treatment of the Offender*. New York: Plenum Press.

Stone, E. (1989). 'Spatial patterns in series of burglaries; an environmental psychological perspective.' Unpublished dissertation, University of Surrey.

Strand, V. (1986). 'Parents in incest families: a study in differences.' Unpublished doctoral dissertation, Columbia University, New York.

Straus, M. A., Kelles, R. J. and Steinmetz, S. K. (1980). *Behind Closed Doors: Violence in the American Family.* New York: Doubleday Anchor.

Strayer, F. F. (1980). 'Social ecology of the preschool peer group.' In Collins, A. (ed.), *Minnesota Symposium on Child Psychology* (volume 13). Hillsdale, NJ: Erlbaum.

Subotnik, L. S. (1989). 'Men who batter women: from overcontrolled to undercontrolled in anger expression.' In Russell, G. W. (ed.) *Violence in Intimate Relationships.* New York: PMA Publishing Corporation.

Suinn, R. M. and Richardson, F. (1971). 'Anxiety management training: a nonspecific behavior therapy program for anxiety control.' *Behaviour Therapy*, 2, 498–510.

Syndulko, K., Parker, D. A., Jens, R., Maltzman, I. and Ziskind, E. (1975). 'Psychophysiology of sociopathy: electrocortical measures.' *Biological Psychology*, 3, 185–200.

Tanner, J. M. (1978). *Fetus into Man: Physical Growth from Conception to Maturity.* Cambridge, MA: Harvard University Press.

Thorndike, E. L. (1932). *The Psychology of Learning.* New York: Teachers College.

Toch, H. (1969). *Violent Men.* Chicago: Aldine.

Toch, H. (ed.) (1979). *Psychology of Crime and Criminal Justice.* New York: Holt Rinehart & Winston.

Toch, H. (1992). *Violent Men; an Inquiry into the Psychology of Violence* (revised edition). Washington DC: American Psychological Association.

Towl, G. J. (1990). 'Understanding the voices.' *Nursing Times*, 86, No 2. London: Macmillan Magazines.

Towl, G. J. (1993). 'Anger control groupwork in practice', In Clark, N. K. and Stephenson, G. M. (eds) *Children, Evidence and Procedure. Issues in Criminological and Legal Psychology*, No 20. Leicester, UK: British Psychological Society.

Towl, G. J. (1994a). 'Anger control: A facilitator's handbook.' HM Prison Service internal publication, London.

Towl, G. J. (1994b). 'Anger control groupwork in prisons.' In Stanko, E. (ed.) *Perspectives on Violence.* London: Howard League Handbooks, Quartet Books Ltd.

Towl, G. J. (1994c). 'Ethical issues in forensic psychology.' *Forensic Update.* Leicester, UK: British Psychological Society.

Towl, G. J. (1995). 'Anger management groupwork.' In Towl, G. J. (ed.) *Groupwork in Prisons, Issues in Criminological and Legal Psychology*, No 24. Leicester, UK: Britsh Psychological Society.

Towl, G. J. and Crighton, D. A. (1995). 'Risk assessment in prisons: a psychological setting.' *Forensic Update*, 40. Leicester, British Psychological Society.

Towl, G. J. and Dexter, P. (1994). 'Anger management groupwork in prisons: an empirical evaluation.' *Groupwork*, Volume 7. London: Whiting & Birch.

Townsend, P. (1993). *The International Analysis of Poverty.* London: Harvester Wheatsheaf.

Townsend, P., Whitehead, M. and Davidson, N. (1992). *Inequality in Health, the Black Report and the Health Divide.* London: Penguin Books.

Truesdell, D. L., McNeil, J. S. and Deschner, J. (1986). 'The incidence of wife abuse in incestuous families.' *Social Work*, March-April, 138–40.

Tumim, S. (1990). *Report of a Review by HM Chief Inspector of Prisons for England and Wales of Suicide and Self-harm in Prison Service Establishments in England and Wales.* London: HMSO.

Turner, S. (1969). 'Delinquency and distance.' In Wolfgang, M. E. and Sellin, T. (eds) *Delinquency: Selected Studies.* New York: Wiley.

Tversky, D. and Kahneman, A. (1974). 'Judgment under uncertainty, heuristics and biases.' *Science,* 185, 1124–31.

Walker, L. J. (1980). 'Cognitive perspective taking prerequisites for moral development.' *Child Development,* 51, 131–9.

Walker, N., Hammond, W. and Steer, D. (1967). 'Repeated violence.' *Criminal Law Review,* 465–72.

Walton, J. M. (1988). 'From private sorrow to public concern? Policy responses to domestic violence in Britain, the United States of America and Sweden.' Dissertation submitted for B Soc Sci in Comparative Social Administration, University of Birmingham, England.

Warr, P. B. (1987). *Work, Unemployment and Mental Health.* Oxford: Oxford University Press.

Watson, J. B. (1913). 'Psychology as the behaviorist views it.' *Psychological Review,* 20, 158–77.

Watson, J. B. and Rayner, R. (1920). 'Conditioned emotional reactions.' *Journal of Experimental Psychology,* 3, 1–14.

Wenk, E., Robinson, J. and Smith, G. (1972). 'Can violence be predicted?' *Crime and Delinquency,* 18, 393–402.

Wicker, A. W. (1969). 'Attitudes versus actions: the relationship of overt and behavioral responses to attitude objects.' *Journal of Social Issues,* 25, 41–78.

Wilson, E. (1983) *What is to be done about Violence against Women?* London: Penguin.

Williams, J. M. G. (1994). *The Psychological Treatment of Depression: A Guide to the Theory and Practice of Cognitive Behaviour Therapy* (2nd editon). London: Routledge.

Williams, L. M. and Finkelhor, D. (1990). 'The characteristics of incestuous fathers.' In Marshall, W. L., Laws, D. R. and Barbaree, H. E. (eds) *Handbook of Sexual Assault: Issues, Theories, and Treatment of the Offender.* New York: Plenum Press.

Wilson, E. (1983) *What is to be done about Violence against Women?* London: Penguin.

Wolfgang, M. E. (1958). *Patterns in Criminal Homicide.* Philadelphia: University of Pennsylvania Press.

Wolfgang, M. E. (ed.) (1967). *Studies in Homicide.* New York: Harper & Row.

Wolfgang, M. E. (1986). 'Homicide in other industrialized countries.' *Bulletin of the New York Academy of Medicine,* 62, 410–12.

Wolfgang, M. E. and Ferracuti, F. (1967). *The Subculture of Violence.* London: Tavistock.

Wolfgang, M. E. and Weiner, N. A. (eds) (1982). *Criminal Violence.* London: Sage Publications.

Wolpe, J. (1958). *Psychotherapy by Reciprocal Inhibition.* Stanford, CA: Stanford University Press.

Woodruffe, C. (1990). *Assessment Centres.* London: Institute of Personnel Management.

Wydra, A., Marshall, W. L., Earls, C. M. and Barbaree, H. E. (1983). 'Identification of cues and control of sexual arousal by rapists.' *Behaviour Research and Therapy*, 21, 469–76.

Yates, E. P., Barbaree, H. E. and Marshall, W. L. (1984). 'Anger and deviant sexual arousal.' *Behavioural Therapy*, 15, 287–94.

Zajonc, R. B. (1980). 'Thinking and feeling: preferences need no inferences.' *American Psychologist*, 35, 151–75.

Zaslow, M. J. and Hayes, C. D. (1986). 'Sex differences in children's responses to psychosocial stress: towards a cross-context analysis.' In Lamb, M. E., Brown, A. L. and Rogoff, B. (eds) *Advances in Developmental Psychology* (Volume 4). Hillsdale, NJ: Erlbaum.

Zimbardo, P. G. (1969). 'The human choice: individuation, reason and order versus deindividuation, impulse and chaos.' In Arnold, W. J. and Levine, K. (eds) *Nebraska Symposium on Motivation*, 17, 237–307.

Zimbardo, P. G. (1975). 'On transforming experimental research into advocacy for social change.' In Deutch, M. and Hornstein, H. (eds) *Applying Social Psychology: Implications for Research, Practice and Training*. Hillsdale, NJ: Lawrence Erlbaum.

Subject index

Name index

Breinigsville, PA USA
16 August 2009
222395BV00003B/25/A